# Dancing with Cancer

by Loui Tucker

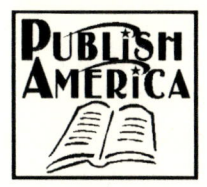

PublishAmerica
Baltimore

© 2004 by Loui Tucker.
All rights reserved. No part of this book may be reproduced, stored in a retrieval system or transmitted in any form or by any means without the prior written permission of the publishers, except by a reviewer who may quote brief passages in a review to be printed in a newspaper, magazine or journal.

First printing

*Photo Credits:*
pages 20-22: photos by Ann Kleiman
page 40: photo by Bruce Meisner
page 47: photo on right by Bruce Meisner; photo on left manipulated with Photoshop by Lee Myers
pages 156-159: photos by David Bergen

ISBN: 1-4137-1587-7
PUBLISHED BY PUBLISHAMERICA, LLLP
www.publishamerica.com
Baltimore

Printed in the United States of America

For the women who walked
this road before me,
and for the women who will follow me.

# INTRODUCTION

I was diagnosed with Stage Two breast cancer in mid-April, 2002. Because it was the easiest, most efficient way to tell *all* of my family members, friends, clients, students, and colleagues at once, without making numerous phone calls, I sent out an e-mail to a few dozen people informing them of the situation.

Over the next few weeks, when I got responses and questions, I wrote individual replies. That quickly became time consuming and I tired of re-writing the same information over and over. I solved that by writing one answer in my word processing software and saving it. When I needed to, I copied and pasted it into an e-mail response. Even that became burdensome, so I set up an e-mail group and began sending out a single update every Sunday night.

Then things really got out of hand. Some recipients began forwarding my weekly e-mail to friends. Those friends then e-mailed me and asked to be added to my e-mail group so they could receive their own e-mail each week. People who heard about the weekly e-mails began handing me business cards and slips of paper with their e-mail address on it and ask to be added to my e-mail list. By August, the number of recipients had nearly tripled and the Sunday reports were going out to nearly 200 e-mail addresses.

By the end of January 2003, the "subscribers" numbered over 250, and the e-mails were being forwarded to many more.

I got a lot of encouragement to write this book. Others wrote:

> I adore your letters… They are so intensely honest and about what is real for you this moment in time… Hope

you don't mind that I'm sharing your e-mails with my older sister. It has occurred to me that you should be keeping all your e-mail messages in a special journal and perhaps think about publishing it for those who are not so articulate....

I hope you don't mind, but I have printed every e-mail you have sent since this journey of yours began and distributed them among my women friends, and the feedback I get is understandingly awesome...by that I mean THEY are awed by your attitude, your writing and most of all by your ability to remain so grounded. One of the comments was "I don't think I've ever known anyone who was so 'right out there.' She keeps it so real." (Maybe Annie Lamott, the author of *Operating Instructions* would come close.) So, keep them coming my dear, we are all listening.

By the way, all of the Internet addresses and websites noted in this book are still accurate. If you want to see the many photos mentioned, they are still posted.

* * * * * * * * * * * *

# I HAVE SOME NEWS, AND IT ISN'T GOOD

## Tuesday, April 23, 2002, 1:30 AM

In mid-March, a mammogram showed an "architectural anomaly." In early April, a follow-up mammogram and ultrasound showed a "suspicious lump." I had surgery last Friday, April 19, and the lump was cancerous, just under 2 cm in diameter. The blood work they did indicates my liver is fine; the chest x-ray showed my lungs are fine. Brain function appears to be normal and I have no bone pain, so the cancer has not spread there. Right now, I feel fine except for being sore where the incision was made.

So what does this mean? Short answer: Breast cancer.

I'll start chemotherapy treatment in mid-May after I have one more surgery to check my lymph nodes (that's this coming Friday, April 26). Even if no lymph nodes show signs of cancer, it still means chemotherapy, but "cautious" chemotherapy. The more lymph nodes are involved, the more aggressive the chemotherapy drug combination. Some chemotherapy is once a week for six months. It's the drug combination that dictates how aggressive it is, not the length of the treatment. Six months from mid-May means until mid-November.

I hope to take the chemotherapy drugs on a Friday so that I'll feel lousy on the weekend but able to function and work and teach my dance classes as I typically do Monday through Friday.

They tell me that most people lose their hair around the second week. That means *all* hair, including eyebrows and eyelashes. Oh, goodie! And when that's over, I get six weeks of daily radiation treatment that I'm told is like having a bad localized sunburn. (And I thought the stress I went through with the treatment for skin cancer two years ago was a bother! Silly me!) By my calculations, this should all be behind me by January, 2003.

However, there is good news: upwards of a 90% cure rate for this type of cancer when caught in the early stages, before the lymph system is involved and the cancer has begun to travel through the body.

## IN SPITE OF ALL THIS, I AM GRATEFUL

- that I live at a time when the medical profession has advanced to the point where I can expect to be cured. As little as 50 years ago, that lump might not have been found until it was too late. I will be inconvenienced, I will suffer side effects, and I may not have the energy and enthusiasm that I (and you) are used to, but I will survive this.

- that I have good medical coverage. My medical care and treatment will not bankrupt me or send me deep into debt.

- that millions of women have already gone through this. There is security in numbers! I don't have to be a trailblazer or a guinea pig.

- that I will have the daily and tenacious support and love of my partner Sabine and the timely support and love of a vast group of family, friends, and colleagues. Many women have to face this alone.

- that I have a strong, healthy body. My body is not additionally compromised by having to deal with, for example, diabetes or lupus.

Now, I ask that all of you reading this help me. Please, do not make this the topic of *every* conversation you have with me. I still have my work, my dance classes, a love of good food and long walks in my neighborhood, a wish for more time to read, a passion for social justice, a home with an 80%-complete remodeled kitchen, and so much more. I know you will care and be concerned, but coddling and fussing are Sabine's job. (And, by the way, Sabine will need your support too.) Your job is to encourage me to smile and laugh, and help me focus on my life and my future.

Thanks, in advance, for being there for me.

Loui

* * * * * * * * * * * * *

# QUICK UPDATE

## Monday, April 29, 2002, 4:00 PM

Update on my medical condition, for those who want to know:

I had surgery last Friday to completely remove the 1.5 cm breast lump (prior surgery was just a biopsy), and take a sample of the lymph tissue under my arm. The sentinel (primary) lymph node tested positive for cancer. The test on the remaining lymph tissue won't be complete until this Friday. That test will indicate what types of drugs will be used in the chemotherapy, which will probably begin the middle of May.

I am sore and bruised where the two incisions were made, and I can feel the annoying lymph drain that has to be left in for a week, but otherwise I feel fine. Really! Sudden arm movements with my left arm and any bouncing, jumping, and hopping cause some discomfort (actually going up is fine; it's the landing that hurts), so I'm going to avoid those kinds of movements for a while. Gentle hugs are not painful.

I am planning on teaching my dance class tonight, Wednesday, and Thursday. I want to dance as much as I can. Sabine says she will be watching me like a hawk to be certain I don't overdue it. I have scheduled myself only half-days of work for right now, so I'll have time to nap if I need to. Shirley volunteered to work with the beginners, teach, and/or be there as backup in the event I'm just too tired and want to sit for a while. Both she and Mark offered assistance if I needed it, which is very reassuring.

I've been receiving an astonishing assortment of jokes since I asked for people to keep me laughing. Here's a favorite:

*Dancing with Cancer*

This guy goes to see a psychiatrist and tries to explain his problem. "I think I'm a dog. I like to chase cars, I wake up and start barking in the middle of the night, and I even have a craving for dog food. Yesterday I tried to scratch my ear with my foot!"

The psychiatrist says, "This is fascinating. I have a lot of experience with these kinds of disorders. Why don't you go lie down over there and we'll start our session."

However, the patient doesn't move.

"What's wrong?" asked the psychiatrist.

The man replied, "I'm not allowed on the furniture."

That's all for now. Thanks for all your care and concern. I am rich in friends!

Loui

* * * * * * * * * * * * *

# LATE-BREAKING NEWS

## Sunday, May 5, 2002, 7:30 PM

I'm doing miles better now that the evil drain has been removed. It was like trying to move, sleep, shower, etc, with a pencil stuck in your armpit! I have full mobility again (thank you!), and I'm just dealing with residual numbness in the armpit and surrounding area. I'm told the numbness will fade with time. I certainly hope so.

The pathology report came back with four lymph nodes testing positive, which means I'm on the very low edge of the guidelines for aggressive chemotherapy (as opposed to cautious or very aggressive). Stage Two breast cancer.

This Tuesday I have an appointment with an oncologist to discuss treatment options. I'll keep you posted....

Loui

* * * * * * * * * * * * *

# ANOTHER UPDATE

## Tuesday, May 7, 2002, 10:15 PM

Some of this may be more information than you need. Feel free to skip what isn't interesting....

I took the pathology report on my lymph nodes to an oncologist today (Tuesday, May 7). Four lymph nodes (out of the 11 they tested) came up positive. Of the four additional factors they tested for (estrogen level and growth rate being two of them), I received three "favorable" readings and one "unfavorable" reading. The oncologist also factors in my age, general health, number of positive nodes, size of the original tumor, relationship to menopause (I'm on the cusp), etc. Then all that gets run through a slick computer model based on data from the hundreds of thousands of women who've been down this road already. It compares me to women with similar ratings, what drug regimen they took and the resulting rate of recurrence of cancer, the severity of the recurrence, mortality, etc. The computer program allows you to try out various drug scenarios and look at the resulting statistical forecasts.

After looking at the top three drug possibilities for my factors, I'm fairly certain I will be using a combination that goes by the letters "CAF"–Cytoxan, Adriamycin, and 5-Fluorouracil. This combination gives me the statistically best chance of not having a recurrence, significantly better than the "CMF" combination, which was the next best choice. CAF is aggressive and has an excellent track record both in the U.S. and Europe.

With the oncologist's approval I will delay chemotherapy until AFTER Memorial Day (I'll be able to attend Rikud Dance Camp in

Simi Valley, California!). He agrees I need to be completely healed from the two surgeries and in the best physical and mental shape possible, because (Newsflash!) chemo is not easy.

I start chemotherapy Friday, May 31. It's a 28-day regime. The morning of Day #1 and Day #8, I'll get a one-hour intravenous drip of the basic nasty stuff. Days #1–#14, I also take another drug orally. Days #14–#27, I recuperate. I do that cycle 6 times, finishing up sometime near the end of November. Then I do six weeks of radiation. But that's waaaay down the road.

My IV drip will also include some wonderful new anti-nausea drugs, and I'm told that if you're in generally good health (as I am), the nausea is minimized if not eliminated. (Otherwise, you're pretty queasy at least for Day #1 and #2 and again Day #8 and #9.)

Day #15–#21, you're reportedly the most tired because you've got the full blast of the drugs in your system. Days #21–#27, you supposedly feel pretty good as your blood and body recuperate from the onslaught, at which point you do it all again!

Somewhere around the second week, 95+% of patients lose their hair, *all* of it. I will not wear a wig! I will not wear false eyelashes! I have a friend designing a henna tattoo for my bald pate, something decorative but with a political message. I haven't decided on the text yet. Perhaps "Chemotherapy at Work." Or "Go Ahead! Ask Me Why I'm Bald!" Okay, okay, I suppose I'll have to wear a scarf or bandana on occasion....

So there we have it. Mr. Toad's Wild Ride is about to begin. Hang on, it's going to be a bumpy ride!

Thanks to *everyone* for all the cards and e-mail and voice-mail and flowers and plants and food and gifts and books and offers of an ear/shoulder. I am blessed with the love and support of so many wonderful friends! I hope to fly through the next six months on the wings of their good thoughts.

Loui

* * * * * * * * * * * *

# BE AMONG THE FIRST TO SEE ME BALD!

## Wednesday, May 16, 2002, 11:40 AM

The chemo's going to take my hair anyway, so I'm going to do a pre-emptive strike and turn the hair loss into a celebration/liberation. Wanna come to the party and watch me take it *ALL* off?

Tuesday, June 4, 2002
6:30 PM
Brian's Back Lot Salon
25 Norton Street (just north of the intersection of San Carlos and Meridian)
San Jose, CA 95126
408-298-8269

I'm gonna supply an assortment of pizzas, sodas, and bottled water. Bring a camera, bring noisemakers, bring your favorite upbeat music. Wear something amusing.

Come help me say hello to my bare scalp!

Loui

* * * * * * * * * * * * *

# STARTING DOWN THE ROAD

## Sunday, June 2, 2002, 5:50 PM

So many of you have already called and e-mailed to check up on me. Thank you for your concern and good wishes. It feels so good knowing so many people are thinking of me, sending me strength and healing. I hope nobody is upset with just receiving a general response. There just isn't time for individual phone calls and responses. I started chemotherapy treatment on schedule May 31, Friday morning, 9:00 AM. It is Sunday evening as I write this.

Actually, things went surprisingly well. The waiting until Friday and not knowing how I was going to react were the hardest part for me (and for Sabine). The actual chemotherapy was rather anti-climactic!

Friday, I felt like nothing had happened. (Really! Details below.) Saturday, I started taking the second drug orally and that made me a tad queasy and lightheaded and thirsty, but I was able to get out and socialize a bit. I slept badly Saturday night and didn't really recover until mid-afternoon Sunday. Right now, I'm just feeling listless, rather like I'm coming down with a cold or the flu. I can tell the nausea's still there because my sense of smell is out of whack, and my appetite is suppressed.

Assuming I'm over the worst of it for the week, I hope to be feeling pretty normal by tomorrow morning.

If that's all you wanted to know, the rest is just details. Read on if you're interested.

The chemo is not administered in a drip line while you sit and read a book, which is what I'd been led to believe would happen. I'm getting that combination of drugs called CAF. Other drug combinations are done with a drip line while you sit and read, but not this one.

With CAF, an RN actually sets up the IV with a bag of saline and then sits next to you and manually adds the bags of liquid drugs to the drip line. There is some concern about "vein pain" with Adriamycin especially because it can cause a burning sensation, so they want to be able to stop administration of the drug immediately if there is a problem. While squeezing out the drugs, the RN chatted away about what the drugs are designed to do, *probable* side effects versus *possible* side effects, what to do in case of an emergency (high fever, diarrhea, etc.), and how to take the oral medications.

So, I had my book to read and my Lifesavers to suck on (for the dry mouth and metallic taste I was told to expect), but I didn't need either one! (Thanks anyway, Cathy!) I've since discovered that if you take the Cytoxan (the "C" in the CAF) in the IV you get the metallic taste in your mouth. If you take it orally, you skip that side effect.

I was told the biggest side effect would be nausea, but the first drug they give you in the IV line is a fairly new nausea fighter called Kytril that must be terrific because Friday I didn't feel even queasy! They also give you a small dose of some steroid that gives you an energy boost for the first 24 hours, to get you over the worst of the Adriamycin and the 5-Fluorouracil. I could have driven home from the treatment (Sabine was with me the whole time for the first visit and took copious notes), and I plan to do so in the future. I was able to eat lunch and dinner, and Friday night I kept my commitment to lead the dancing at Shir Hadash after Friday night services.

The Adriamycin and 5-FU (such an accurate nickname for 5-Fluorouracil) circulate in your system for about 48 hours and then you're down to just dealing with the Cytoxan. Because of a mix-up at the pharmacy I had to wait until Saturday morning to start the oral Cytoxan.

The Kytril is great against nausea, but its side effect is killer constipation. We're talking cement! Lots of water and milk of magnesia do a pretty good job against that. It's kind of a crazy chain reaction—a problem gets solved by a drug, which causes a side effect, which is solved by another drug, which creates a side effect...and so on until you get to a side effect you can live with.

I'll be getting my head shaved this Tuesday the 4th. No, I'm not going for just a Marine-style buzz haircut. It might as well all come off now so I can start getting used to it. Lots of people are bringing cameras to the Grooming Party on Tuesday, so I'll send out "before" and "after" photos later in the week. (If you didn't get an official invitation, please e-mail me, and I'll send you the particulars.) The chemo will take the stubble and remaining body hair off during the weeks ahead. If you have stories for me about acquaintances, friends, and relatives who didn't lose their hair, you don't need to tell me. They were probably taking the CMF regimen. The "M" in CMF is similar to Adriamycin, not quite as strong, and only effects hair growth in about 30% of the patients. On the other hand, something below 2% of the patients taking Adriamycin manage to keep any hair. Adriamycin's sole job is to kill fast-growing cells. Cancer cells grow quickly (double approx. once every 100 days), but so does your hair and mucous membrane, and since Adriamycin can't tell the difference between a good fast-growing cell and a bad one, it just kills them all.

So, this will be my life for a while. Two weeks of chemo and two weeks to rest up for the next round. Six rounds. Sigh.... Again, Sabine and I both send big grateful thank yous to everyone!

Loui

* * * * * * * * * * * * *

# THE LIBERATION OF MY SCALP

Sunday, June 9, 2002, 8:24 PM

The head-shaving party was terrific! Over fifty loving supporters, some in crazy costumes, consuming pizza and champagne, packed into a small hair salon, spilling onto the balcony and front lawn. There was so much energy and love reverberating from the walls that it was impossible for me to feel scared or sad or tired.

So many brought crazy gifts. I got a blond wig from David Bergen (who loves to remind me that, back in 1975, he happened to take a photo of me when I wore my hair long and bleached blond). I got candles and CDs and bottles of sunscreen, and a silly crown and a magic wand, and t-shirts, and a really nice embroidered hat, and balloons and cards and bouquets of flowers! Ovi Saenz, a local professional photographer, presented Sabine and me with a framed copy of a picture he'd taken of us all dressed up for Oscar Night back in March, back when I had hair and this cancer thing was weeks away in my future! Ann Kleiman made commemorative badges for all to wear that said: "There is nothing, nothing, nothing that two women cannot do before noon."

A big thank you goes to Brian Finney for opening his Back Lot Studio to me and all the madness. I still marvel at Brian and Robert who (with some help from Rich) managed to do *eleven* heads (two complete shaves, several very, very short cuts, and three just short haircuts) in just over three hours, and all while a wild party raged around them. Not one ear was nicked…. What concentration!

And the event actually made the local evening and early morning news! No kidding! Another client of the salon, who is a reporter at the local NBC affiliate, heard about the party from Brian, asked for permission to attend, shoot some footage, and interview participants. My 30 seconds of fame, and I'm bald! Yikes!

I've only had time to put up six quick photos. Go to: www.louitucker.com/photos.htm

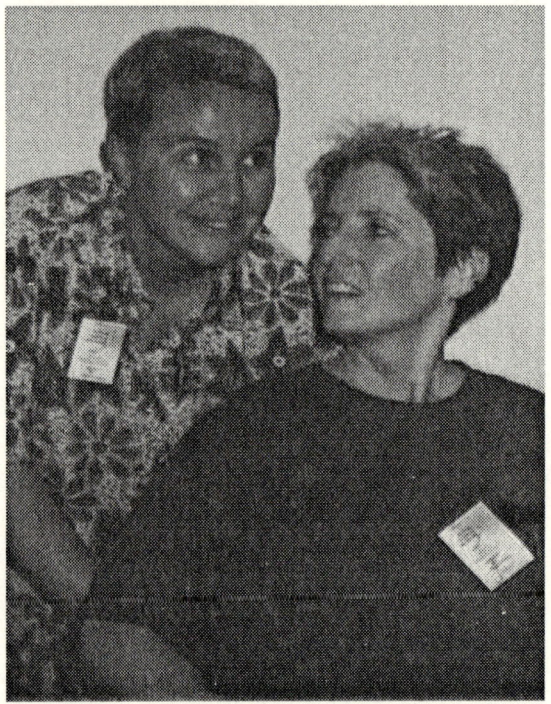

*Before the shave*

## MISC. THOUGHTS ON BEING SUDDENLY BALD

Perhaps it's California, perhaps it's our highly tolerant, politically correct culture, or maybe we've gotten so used to green Mohawks and pierced eyebrows and obscenity-emblazoned t-shirts that a woman having no hair on her head is just another fashion statement.

*Dancing with Cancer*

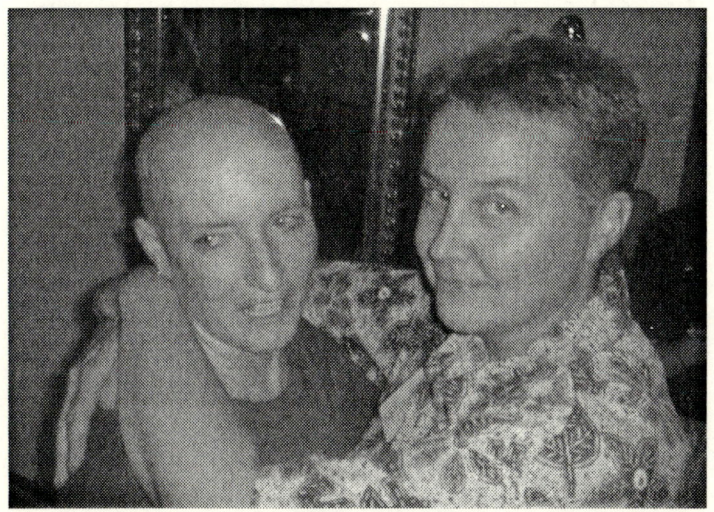

*After the shave*

    Strangers don't even blink! The guy at the gas station hands me my change like he sees bald women in there all the time. I have not stopped a single restaurant conversation mid-sentence. Nobody has turned to stare and consequently walked into a light pole. I have not caused a single traffic accident because a driver did a double-take on the freeway. No child in a supermarket has shrieked and hidden behind the leg of a nearby parent at the sight of me. Amazing!
    If you have no hair, and you wake up in the morning, or from a nap, you don't have to worry about having bed hair.
    You lose a LOT of heat through your head. In an air-conditioned office where everyone else is comfortable, my head is cold! I can understand why cartoons depict grandpas wearing a stocking cap to bed! Beyond that, the second round of chemo was a bit tougher than the first. I've been a bit more queasy and tired, and my mouth is always dry. Keep the good thoughts streaming my way....

Loui

* * * * * * * * * * * * *

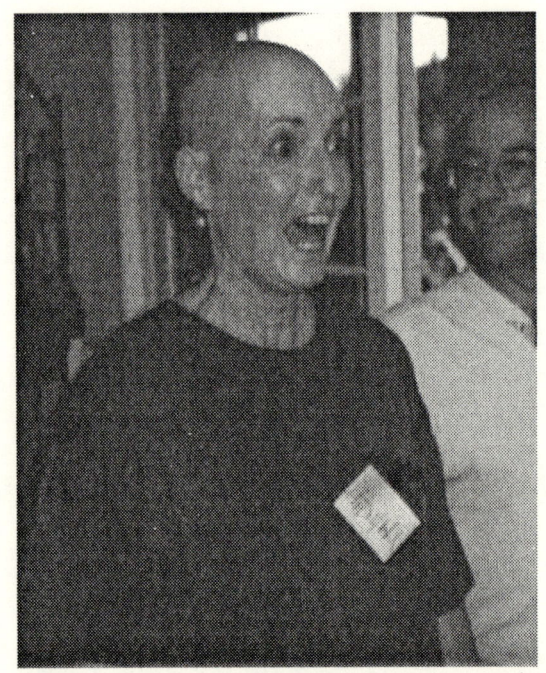

*Oh my God!*

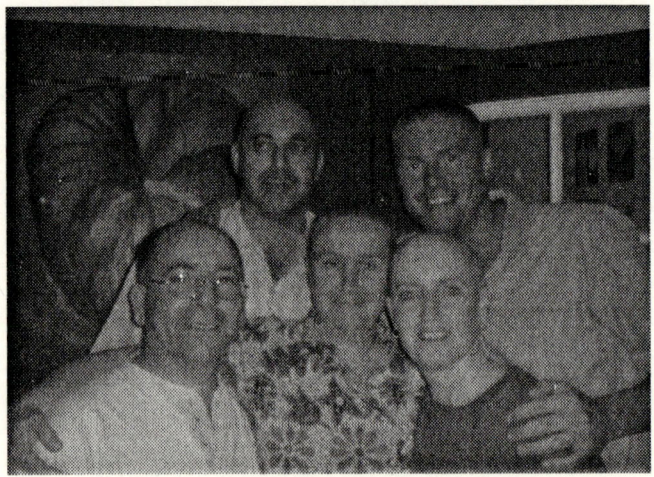

*Group of shaved heads*

# ONE DOWN, FIVE TO GO

## Sunday, June 16, 2002, 10:30 PM

The good news is the first round of chemotherapy ended Friday. I now have two weeks to recuperate, recover, rebound, rebuild, replenish (all those "re-" words) before the next round. I survived. One down, five to go.

I was able to work a pretty full week, considering I get a later start each morning because I can't seem to go from bed-to-shower-to-my-usual-fifth-gear in 30 minutes like I used to. I also need to at least be horizontal (if not actually nap) for an hour in the afternoon. Thank goodness I'm an independent contractor and can set my own hours!

I was able to run my three nights of dance classes, though I was pretty pooped by 11:00 PM on Monday and Wednesday, and I skipped all the usual after-dance gatherings. Dance has always brought me joy, and the endorphin rush is a powerful mood-lifter and pain-killer. I get lots of love and hugs and energy from my dance community. Thank you!

Gifts and treats: I was also treated to a wonderful massage. A member of the Kinsey Sicks (the world's only "dragcapella beauty shop quartet"!) presented me with their latest CD, which had me laughing for an hour! I received a clever and funny, hand-made card from two now-grownup girls I had in dance class, let me think a minute, 15 years ago? The card included a photos of the two of them, then and now, and one of me I'd never seen from (I'm guessing) the mid-1980s. The photo shows me still dancing barefoot and using a *record player*...!

*Loui Tucker*

## THE NOT-SO-GOOD PART OF THE WEEK

The side effects got pretty bad as the week progressed, and it turns out there was a reason. It started with a very dry mouth and a small lump in my throat, which made swallowing uncomfortable. The dry mouth was expected since the chemo drugs wipe out mucous membrane. I coped by sucking on ice cubes.

The visit to the oncologist on Wednesday produced prescriptions for two special mouthwashes. The staff said the washes would take a while to fix things, so I tried to be patient. There was no improvement by Friday. In fact, conditions had deteriorated. My mouth had sores, the lump in my throat was larger, and my tongue felt swollen. I tasted like an old rusty tin can, eating and swallowing were actually painful, and everything tasted rather gray.

**STOMACH**: Yo, HQ! We ain't got no raw materials in the last five hours. How we are supposed to produce the building supplies they've been asking for, huh? Think you could find out what's the problem?

**BRAIN**: One moment please...(muzak while on hold)... The appetite and taste buds are out of commission, and the rest of the system is in bad repair. I'm going to send in a negotiator to see if we can produce some action.

**WILL TO SURVIVE**: Okay, I understand you're under a bit of stress, but the manifests show we've already tapped the reserves all that we dare this week. We've got to get the raw materials past your roadblock.

**MOUTH**: No, negative, nyet, nein, uh-uh, forget it. Not gonna happen.

*Dancing with Cancer*

**WILL TO SURVIVE**: How about something cool and smooth and soft? Come on, you can do it. We can't repair the damage without new supplies. You've gotta help us out here....

So, I was down to cool fruit smoothies, applesauce, avocados, scrambled eggs, and Ensure drinks (thanks to Rich and David for that tip!). Thursday night had me in tears.

**SABINE** (hugging me, trying to boost my spirits): "Hey, you got through the first treatment. One down, just five to go."

**ME**: "Five to go? Five more months of this??? I can't believe I'm going to feel like this for five more months! July, August, September, October, November.... Waaaah!"

Friday meant another trip to the oncologist for a blood test. While waiting for the results, the nurse chatted about diet and dealing with the mouth sores. The test came back. The nurse took one look at it and said, "Hmm. I need to see the doctor," and walked away. Well! What did that mean?

She came back with the news that, lo and behold, I had ZERO white blood cells! ZERO! Actually, I think I had two left (Maude and Ralph), and they were too busy mounting an attack in my mouth to show up for the test. It appears that, while my immune system was depressed from all the chemo drugs, an opportunistic infection had moved into my mouth like a bunch of thugs into a poorly policed neighborhood and were causing all the havoc.

I got a prescription for a kick-ass antibiotic and a terrific mouthwash called (write this one down) "The Stanford

Mouthwash." It's some formula the Stanford doctors concocted and has to be mixed by a compounding pharmacist (not just a pill dispenser), and kept refrigerated. And, of course, being not-a-brand-name-or-generic drug, it's not covered by insurance. No problem. This stuff works, and it's worth the $60. That and the antibiotic went to the rescue of the beleaguered but valiant Maude and Ralph, and I was already feeling better Friday afternoon. Not great, but vastly improved. Saturday and Sunday, I actually ate carefully chewed real food, and my taste buds have gradually recovered. I'll check in with the oncologist Monday for another blood test and see if my white blood cell count has risen sufficiently. If not, they promised yet another drug to prod my bone marrow into producing more white blood cells.

Now, did you need to know all that? I don't know, but I do know it helps me to write this all down each week. I found years ago that, whether I'm reporting on a meeting or conference I've attended or sharing a personal crisis with a friend through correspondence, writing is awesome therapy. The process of analyzing, organizing, and describing, and getting it out of my head and onto paper (or computer screen) transfers the event from active memory to storage and I can focus forward again. If the event has painful emotional tags attached to it, the humor, whether I can find it in the situation or have to inject it myself, seems to remove the tag. Making myself smile while I write this, and thinking that perhaps you smiled as you read this, is good therapy too.

To close, I have one more request, folks, especially of you who dance in one of my three classes. My immune system is compromised right now and I'm highly vulnerable to infections. If you have a cold or flu symptoms, please, *please* stay home from dance class. I promise I'll miss you, but it's important to me that you not come near me. The bacteria and germs can be passed from hand to hand and on to me and will make me very sick, very quickly. My body has enough to do killing marauding cancer cells right now. I (as well as Maude and Ralph) will appreciate it!

As the e-mail list grows, I know the positive thoughts flowing my way increase. Thanks for all the little things so many of you do for me. Thanks for being there.

Loui

* * * * * * * * * * * * *

# MAUDE AND RALPH HAVE FRIENDS!

## Sunday, June 23, 2002, 11:15 PM

When we last looked in on Maude and Ralph, they were firing salvos into the nasty thugs that had invaded my mouth. They got reinforcements last weekend and I am feeling sooo much better!

|  | White blood cells |
|---|---|
| Friday May 31 (start of chemotherapy) | 7.2 (million I suppose?) |
| Friday June 7 (second week of chemo) | 5.4 |
| Friday June 14 (third week–no chemo) | zero |
| Thursday, June 20 checkup | 2.9 |

Last week I got some shots of Neupogen, which encouraged my bone marrow to increase production of white blood cells. It's an odd sensation to be standing talking to someone and you feel your pelvic bone throb rather noticeably for about 10 seconds (pushing out white blood cells, or so I'm told). That happened periodically as the bones responded to the Neupogen. It appears to have worked, since the WBC went up to about 40% of where they need to be in less than a week. And although the white blood cell numbers are going back up, the overall numbers say I'm still anemic (red blood cells are down).

So this is the fourth week in the cycle. No chemo, no pills, no shots. My appetite and taste buds are back and so's most of my energy. They keep saying I should feel fatigue. That's not exactly what I call it. It's stamina I don't have. When I need or want to do something, I can. I just run out of steam sooner. It's as if I used to have a 12-gallon gas tank and now I'm been reduced to just 10 gallons. Same fuel efficiency, same speeds possible, just not the same distance on a single tank. But I'm not complaining! I feel fine right now and anticipate having a terrific week.

By the way, I had to tell several people last week: No, I did not feel any pain at all from the cancer before it was discovered. The lump in my breast was found during a routine mammogram. Unlike other cancers that invade and inhibit the functioning of an organ (pancreas, brain, lung, liver), breast cancer pretty much just sits there. Unless it gets very big or you do regular breast exams, you don't know it's there. Even when the cancer sneaks off into the lymph nodes, you're not aware of it. Which brings me to my message:

**EARLY DETECTION IN BREAST CANCER IS VITAL!**

Here are some interesting numbers: A single cancer cells will reproduce itself about once every 100 days. So 1 cell becomes 2 cells, becomes 4 cells, becomes 8 cells in about a year. Insignificant. Then 8 become 16 become 32 become 64 the second year. Still microscopic. But as time passes you have 1,000 becoming 2,000 becoming 4,000 becoming 8,000 and so forth. Yes, there are fast-growing cancers, but the *average* cancer can take 8 years to grow to something the size of grain of rice. That's when things get dicey: 100 days later you have 2 grains of rice, and 100 *more* days and you have 4 grains of rice. Something the size of four grains of rice can be spotted on a mammogram and eight grains of rice can easily be felt. By my calculations, my 1.5 cm lump probably started growing in the early to mid-1990s.

Which leads me to this: if you're a woman, schedule yourself for a mammogram as soon as possible and get them at least once a year after that. Laugh at the bad jokes, wince at the discomfort, but get it done. That lump the size of 4 grains of rice that you cannot feel can be real trouble if it doubles or quadruples while you're putting off that mammogram until next year. If that cancer has a chance to invade your lymph nodes, you'll be traveling down the road I'm currently taking and I don't think you want that!

If you're a man, it's remotely possible you could get breast cancer, but you should first see to it that every woman who is important to you in your life schedules that mammogram.

Again, the trick in treating breast cancer is to catch it early. Breast cancer is survivable, but the cure is not fun. The larger the lump, the more lymph nodes are involved, the less fun it will be.

To end on a lighter note: Sabine and I decided to go to a local soccer game on Saturday. We were standing in line to buy tickets, along with dozens of other soccer fans. A man approached us, handed us two tickets and said, "Here are two tickets to the game. I can't use them. I don't want them to go to waste. Can you use them?" How about that! Just picked us out of the line and there we were with two free passes to the game! See, I told you it was going to be a good week!

Friday, June 28, I start Round Two. Ding!

Loui

* * * * * * * * * * * * *

# ROUND TWO

## Monday July 1, 2002, 10:00 AM

Last week (Monday-Saturday) was actually pretty terrific. I recovered nicely and had lots of energy and a good appetite. The chemotherapy on Friday the 28th was fine. The doctor decided to lower the overall dosages about 10% to give Maude and Ralph a fighting chance this month. Friday and Saturday were fine. I was able to socialize and was feeling confident and strong.

Then came Sunday. Those of you who have written to say I am a source of inspiration would not have found me particularly inspiring on Sunday. I felt like I had the flu: weak and queasy, with a headache, and my tongue felt like a wad of cotton in my mouth. I slept close to 15 out of 24 hours. That meant I went to bed Saturday night, got up and had breakfast and did the *Sunday Times* crossword puzzle with Sabine, went back to bed for two hours, got up and showered, did the grocery shopping, and went back to bed for two hours. I got up one more time to read e-mail, and went back to bed for an hour. And I wasn't just resting, I was sleeping all that time!

Which meant I didn't get this written as I usually do on Sunday night, and I'm sorry if I worried anyone. Monday, as I write this, I'm doing much better. Thankfully I had my Monday client cancel so I don't have to go rushing off to work downtown.

## SOME GOOD THINGS THAT HAPPENED

I continue to receive wonderful e-mails and cards and phone messages. It amazes me that one person who knows me tells someone else what is going on, who tells a third person, who tells a fourth person, and then I get this e-mail from someone I haven't heard from in years!

On the humorous side, my hair continues to vacate my body. The stubble that grew back after I shaved my head three weeks ago is gradually falling out. If I stand over the sink and rub my head briskly with my hand, the surface of the sink quickly shows little black bits of hair. One underarm has hair, but the other does not. I still have my eyebrows and eyelashes, which is a good thing!

## SELF-ESTEEM BOOSTER, PART ONE

On the medical side, I agreed to participate in a study at the oncology clinic that is looking at a drug that has proven effective in fighting kidney-disease-related anemia. They want to determine if it will be equally effective in dealing with chemotherapy-related anemia. Because my red blood cell count is low but I am not reporting great fatigue, they thought I would be a good subject.

The test involves some shots of the drug and both subjective and objective testing. The subjective test is a questionnaire covering perceived and reported fatigue. Some patients have good red blood cell counts and report wicked fatigue. Others, like me, have low red blood cell counts and report minimal or light fatigue.

The stress test was both interesting and validating. They have you do this "step up, step down" test with about an 8" rise for three minutes at a rather slow pace. If that doesn't get your heart rate up to 110, they make you rest and do it again at a slightly higher pace. You are all thinking, "Loui does 3-4 high-energy dances in a row at dance class, so this should be easy." It was easy! I just topped out at 118 after the second 3-minute trial, and still felt fine, glowing but not sweating. Very good for my self-esteem!

## SELF-ESTEEM BOOSTER, PART TWO

On the psychological side, the other nice thing I did for myself I will recommend to anyone who has to do the bald thing. If you know someone who's dealing with cancer treatment, suggest it to them: have some photographs taken! I didn't do the Sears or J.C. Penney thing. I wanted something more than "You have your choice of 6 backgrounds and 7 poses. We'll take 20 shots. You pick the one you like the best and we give you a bunch of copies for $39.99."

I hired Bruce Meisner, a local photographer whose work I've admired. (Visit www.bmeisner.com if you want to see some of his work.) He comes to your house with his equipment, which means if you want to try different clothing, use props, or play with your pets, you can do it. He talks to you about your goals and vision for the photographs. I wanted something artistic, shadowy, serious, beautiful, something that would show the lines and curves of my skull (and Sabine's, since her hair is still very short from the near-shaving three weeks ago). Because Bruce uses a digital camera, we could see the results immediately and make adjustments in lighting and poses. I was so amazed by my appearance.

I have heard and read from many of you that I look good bald and that I have a nicely shaped head, but I had not been able to internalize that message. It took me a week before I stopped being startled by my own reflection in the mirror, and another week before I could accept what I saw as "this is what I look like now." Whatever confidence and self-assurance you saw in me was sheer bravado and willpower.

Having seen Bruce's photographs, I can now honestly smile as I take myself out in the world with pride. I *do* look pretty damn good as a bald woman! Once Sabine and I have picked out the best shots and purchased them, I'll post some on my website for you to see for yourself.

*Loui Tucker*

## I HAD A DREAM

Lastly, on the spiritual side, I want to share a wonderful "vision" I had recently, an image that has been a powerful companion the past few days. I was resting one afternoon and saw myself in the center of a concentric circle of my friends and family. The innermost circle had Sabine and her family and my sister and my closest friends. Each concentric circle beyond contained more people—friends, dancers in my classes, lawyers and legal staff with whom I've worked, e-mail friends, and all the people who've asked to receive these e-mails as a way of staying in touch. The circles seemed to go out infinitely, beyond where I could actually focus and distinguish individual faces.

The circles pulsed and throbbed with energy and support, streaming inward toward me in the center, like the reverse of a pebble being dropped into a body of water. Every time I bring up this image, I can feel those waves of healing and support and strength moving inward, leaving me deliciously awash in love and light and courage.

Thank you all, again and again, for being on the other end of these e-mails. This could not have happened even a few years ago. The concept of sharing so quickly and easily with so many, short of printing and mailing a weekly newsletter, would be impossible without the world-shrinking power of e-mail.

Sending love to all of you in my circle(s) of friends.

Loui

* * * * * * * * * * * * *

# WHEN LIFE GIVE YOU LEMONS

## Sunday, July 7, 2002, 5:00 PM

There's that saying "When life give you lemons, make lemonade." Fine, but what if you don't have sweetener or water? You learn to deal with the lemons.

That about sums up my situation when it comes to my mouth and taste buds. The doctor and nurses have confirmed that the dry mouth and diminished sense of taste are going to be the status quo for the next five months, with some improvement during the two weeks I'm not actively taking the chemo drugs. Chemo drugs attack fast-growing cells. Chemo drugs are stupid and cannot tell the difference between a bad fast-growing cell (cancer) and a good fast-growing cell (hair, taste bud, mucous membrane). I'm doing fine without hair, I don't think about it much at all any more, but I am really starting to miss my mouth. Memo to cancer researchers: Make chemo drugs smarter, will ya?

Dry skin? Apply a cream. Dry eyes? Eye drops. Dry hair? Conditioner. Dry mouth? All the websites and cancer-help books and chat rooms say the same thing: cope with it.

What's it like? It's like have a dried-out sponge for a tongue. I drink/sip water constantly, and my mouth never feels moist unless I hold the liquid in my mouth. I don't have enough saliva to lick an envelope. Humans supposedly have something like 10,000 taste buds. I feel like I'm down to a few dozen. Okay, I'm grateful, really and truly grateful, I don't have the mouth sores and thrush I had last month (thanks to The Stanford Mouthwash's daily vigilance), but geees!

And it's all so unpredictable! I used to drink lots of tea, mostly strong and caffeinated, and I think I've had perhaps four mugs of tea in the last six weeks. I just can't taste it.

I could hardly pass the candy jar in the offices where I work without pawing through it for one of those mini-Milky Ways or Three Musketeers. Now candy has no appeal. Hot chocolate, however, is delicious, and I used to consume maybe three cups per year!

> Potatoes: fried is out, but mashed is good
> Eggs: hard boiled—nope; scrambled or over easy—yep!
> Bread: bleah!
> Pancakes, waffles, French toast: yummy!
> Vegetables: only in soup, though salads become okay in the two off-weeks
> Rice: same as vegetables
> Pasta: fine, if in a creamy sauce
> Fruit: mostly okay, if soft and not too tart
> Jello, pudding, applesauce: nice!
> Anything crunchy, crisp, or salty: forget it

Getting enough protein is a problem. I was not a strict vegetarian before starting chemo, but now I can hardly stand to chew, much less swallow, any meat. It has to be very small soft pieces in soup. I add soy protein to milkshakes and smoothies. I also make the standard recipe for Jell-O and add an eight-ounce chunk of tofu in a blender, which produces something pudding-like that's loaded with protein.

My current big worry is that the tomatoes ripening on our vines are going to be wasted on me and my poor remaining taste buds. One of my favorite summer salads is chopped fresh tomatoes, fresh mozzarella in small cubes, fresh basil, a bit of S&P, a drizzle of olive oil. Occasionally I add cubes of avocado. Fabulous! What if I can't taste it?

## LEARNING LIFE'S LESSONS

In my senior year of high school, we had an assignment to finish the sentence: "Life is…." Our teacher must have been trying to stem "senior-itis" by asking us to get serious about what we were going to be doing next.

I remember one of the essays impressed me enough for me to write down in my journal the opening line: "Life is not a lot different from school. It's a series of lessons and tests." The rest of the essay went on to discuss boring lessons and challenging lessons, pop quizzes, relationship seminars, work-related projects, preparing for the big exams, etc., just expanding on the first line.

That essay means more to me every day now. Cancer and chemotherapy are presenting me with very challenging lessons, and there are nearly daily tests.

I'm learning to pay close attention to my body and the signals it sends. If any pain ratchets up a notch or two above normal, it's time to call or visit the nurses at the oncology clinic.

I'm learning not to eat by the clock, but when I'm hungry and food sounds appetizing.

I'm learning to *really* appreciate the days, even hours, when I'm feeling healthy.

I'm learning that writing, working on projects for my clients, and engaging my brain with engrossing movies and books all serve to take my mind off the various whining signals coming from my body.

I'm learning that exercise (in my case dancing) means endorphins and endorphins are both a pain-reliever and a mood-enhancer. (Okay, okay, I knew that before, I'm just confirming it and rejoicing in it.)

I'm learning that an hour spent napping can mean as much as six more hours of energy.

I'm learning that my normal body temperature is not the 98.6 that the textbooks say it should be. Normal for me is about 96.2, and 98.6 means I'm running slight fever.

I'm learning that friendships are the sunshine of life.

*Loui Tucker*

## TREATS THIS WEEK

    Sabine and I invited a small group of friends over for July 4 fix-em-yourself tacos and mixed-fruit shortcake. What with the kitchen remodel, the building of a patio cover, and my chemo treatments, we hadn't had any guests over for months. It was lovely to sit around laughing, sharing stories, and telling jokes. After everyone left, Sabine and I dashed to a spot where we could see the local fireworks display. We shared a street corner with a Latino family and enjoyed all the lights and action while being far enough away to avoid the auditory impact.
    We got to spend part of Friday and Saturday at a beach house south of Santa Cruz, on loan from generous friends. This was not just a little cottage, mind you, but a full-sized two-story house that's a three-minute walk to cliffs overlooking the beach, with another 10 minutes required to get down the cliff to the beach itself. We got in one walk in the afternoon into dusk, plus another the next morning after breakfast. A sweet, sweet memory!
    I'm also being treated to regular massages. I had been getting massages every few weeks for the past couple of years, but now a wonderful dear friend is covering the cost while I'm on chemo. Massages are a pleasure all by themselves, but receiving them as a gift adds another layer of goodness. I get one massage the Thursday just before I start the two weeks on chemo, to get myself ready, and then reward myself with another one on the Thursday I take the last dose of Cytoxan (this Thursday!).
    This Sunday was not as bad a last Sunday (I think). I still slept a lot, but I got it all in before noon and have been up since then, instead of the up-and-down thing I did last Sunday.
    So I'm just four days away from the end of Round Two. I'll have two weeks to re-grow a few thousand taste buds. And, in just one month, I'll be almost half way through!

                                                   Loui

\* \* \* \* \* \* \* \* \* \* \* \* \*

# IT'S BEEN A MIXED WEEK

### Sunday, July 14, 2002, 8:00 PM

Welcome to my Sunday Night Therapy Session. I hope this does you as much good as it does me.

## MARK YOUR CALENDAR AND PLAN TO ATTEND

Saturday night, January 11, 2003, 6:00 PM until midnight. I've already rented the Sunnyvale Community Center Ballroom, where I hold my Monday night dance class, and I'm planning "The Light at the End of the Tunnel" party. If everything goes according to schedule, I'll be celebrating the end of six months of chemotherapy and the requisite month of radiation. I may not have much hair back, but what the heck! It will be catered by the fabulous Shazan Catering (Girls, don't even think of telling me you have a conflict!), decorated with balloons and balloon animals by Twistin' Shout Balloons (you'll be there, won't you?), and there will be music, music, music and dancing, dancing, dancing. Maybe commemorative party favors (Cathy, help me on this one). Maybe I'll even let some strong, burly people hoist me up in a chair and parade me around the room....

## DRY MOUTH

Thanks to several people for their tips on products to reduce dry mouth. It appears they do make and market products for Chemo-

Mouth. The two products I've tried so far are good for about 15 minutes. Not great, but sometimes just the lift I need. It would be nice, though, to have a product that lasts all night so I don't wake up with the sensation that I'm trying to peel my tongue off the roof of my mouth.

## MORE PHOTOS

Use this to see the photos Bruce Meisner took a couple of weeks ago: www.louitucker.com\MeisnerPhotos.htm

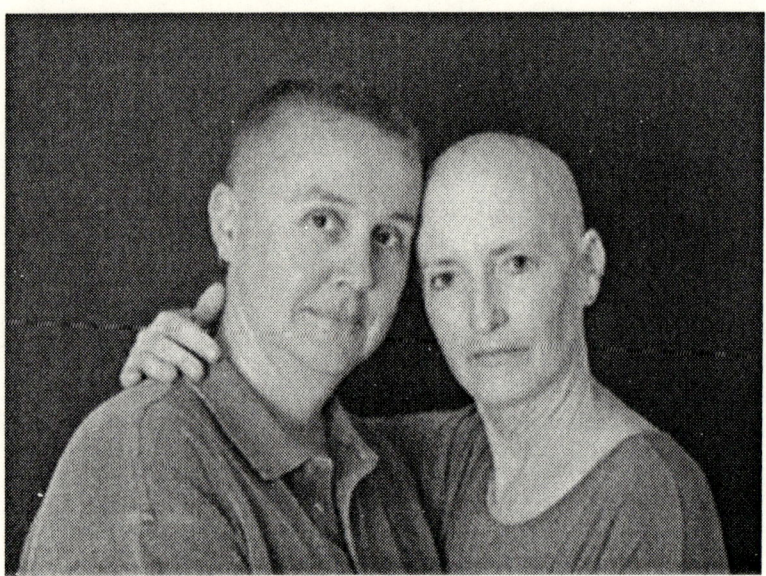

*The two of us*

## YOU ONLY MISS THE WATER WHEN THE WELL RUNS DRY

Another adage for another lesson. I *really* miss my mouth! You who are reading this probably never think much about your tongue and what it does for you. I know I pretty much took mine for granted. Your tongue just sort of lies there in your mouth, useful for moving food around, cleaning gums and teeth, and flapping about when talking. Well, when your tongue goes south, you'll realize how nice it is to have one that doesn't give you grief.

Up through Tuesday, I was pretty much okay, just dealing with the dry mouth. Wednesday morning I woke up thinking someone had snuck into our house that night and done oral surgery on me without my knowledge or consent. I thought surely someone had removed my tongue (which was pretty dried out as it was, but still functioning) and replaced it with something nasty, perhaps a baboon's tongue, or at least from some animal that had a diet of bugs and beetles. At the base, where they'd attached my new tongue, the stitches hurt like the dickens, and they'd left a piece of adhesive bandage dangling down the back of my throat to catch anything that went by. Aaargh! Back to the oncology clinic. Blood tests showed Maude and Ralph still had a few thousand friends, but I once again had sores, this time at the base of my tongue and in my throat. They put me back on an antibiotic and started another round of daily shots of Neupogen to stipulate my bone marrow to make more white blood cells.

I can tell you that when the base of your tongue is sore, it hurts to talk, and my ability in that area is well-known. It really cramps my style when I'm reduced to sign language (Helen, Robin, Jeb and Jory—you would have been proud!) and whispering.

Then Thursday night, *The Slime* showed up! The Slime first appeared as I drank some hot chocolate, and it has not gone away for three loooong days. It feels like my hard palate is coated with a combination of olive oil and Elmer's glue. It's slimy and it won't come off! Not mouthwash, not toothpaste, not food, not cotton swabs—nothing removes The Slime! It's tasteless (thank heavens!), and it doesn't even show up on a cotton swab, but it's waaaaay annoying! Does lymph fluid drip through the roof of your mouth when there's healing to be done??? Each night I go to sleep hoping in the morning it will disappear as mysteriously as it appeared. I'm going to be at the clinic Monday morning for another blood test, and I'll see if anyone knows anything about it or how to get rid of it.

It was encouraging that the doctor admitted this all was an indication he was still giving me too high a dose of the chemo drugs. He assured me that, if the dosages are right, one may have a dry mouth but not the mouth sores. He plans to reduce the dosage yet again this next month. Nice to know this might be the last time I'll have to deal with this particular problem.

On the bright sides, which is to say, above my lips and below my Adam's apple, I'm doing fine! Despite being unable to talk on Thursday, I danced up a full-body sweat. If my energy level used to be like a blow torch, I'm reduced now to being a couple of boxes of matches, but when I want a fire, those matches work just fine, thank you!

My work during the day is reduced, but I'm still out there daily, meeting with clients, running around town massaging software and browbeating computers and printers into doing my bidding.

## TREATS THIS WEEK

Vickie treated us to a movie. She's officially retired, but works part time as a ticket-taker at a local movie house and offered us free tickets any time we wanted. Sabine and I took her up on it and saw *The Divine Secrets of the Ya-Ya Sisterhood*. We'd both read the book, knew what to expect, and still enjoyed it, tears and all.

I treated myself to *Hard Eight* in hardback. This is the eighth book in a series by Janet Evanovich. I put all my pending work aside and I read it cover to cover in two long sittings. I actually laughed out loud several times. I've read the first seven books in the series, so knew I would enjoy it. It was a Saturday well spent! If you're thinking of reading this book yourself, I recommend starting with the first book, *One for the Money*, and go from there. Thank you, Janet Evanovich, wherever you are, and I hope #9 is out soon!

### WORDS TO LIVE BY

Last week I was complaining about losing most of my taste buds. Nicole wrote back: "I'm not sure if it helps, but I wanted to remind you of one fact of life: Whether their taste buds are working or not, many people have no taste at all!" Thank you, Nicole, I needed that!

I also got a great card back near the beginning of all this, but remembered it particularly this weekend: (Outside) "They say you learn the most from your most difficult experiences." (Inside) "What a stupid system." Amen to that!

### A LITTLE BLACK HUMOR ON THE SUBJECT OF WEIGHT LOSS (please try to understand....)

I'm surprised some quack entrepreneur out there hasn't figured out a way to market cancer drugs as part of a diet plan.

> "Need to lose that tummy bulge? Perhaps you'd like to peel a few pounds off each thigh? Want to fit into that little black dress in time for your high school reunion? Fifteen pounds in six weeks? No problem! This newly discovered combination of drugs allows you to eat *anything you want* and still shed those unwanted pounds. No exercise, no special foods, just two little pills. Call toll free today 1-800-xxx-xxxx or visit our website: www.takepoundsoffchemically.com."

The drugs come with a few side effects that they don't tell you about until the package arrives: "Possible side effects: (1) Hair loss—probably all of it—but buy a nice wig for the reunion, you'll look fine; and (2) your taste buds will vacate the premises, and your appetite will go too, with mouth sores moving in while they are gone. We said you could eat anything you wanted, but that's because you won't *want* to eat anything anyway! Hey, you do want to fit into that little black dress, don't you?"

Okay, okay, enough. I'm just a little disturbed about losing 10% of my body weight. I spent too much of my adolescence being underweight and flat-chested, and coveting curves. At the rate I'm going, I'll be back in that space in just a few more months, and that makes me anxious. I know I can gain it all back when this is over, and enjoy every mouthful, but they also assured me that, with the modern drugs, *most* patients do not lose weight during chemotherapy.

Besides, I feel like I need every pound of me, every molecule of me, to be strong and fight this battle, and losing 10% of the troops, even if they are the reserves, will make fighting 10% more difficult.

## FOOD FOR THE FUTURE

To brighten my spirits, which have been flagging the last few days, I've started a list of all the yummies I plan to enjoy the first chance I get.

Nachos with everything on them. Cheese, beans, tomatoes, sour cream, guacamole, onions, the works!

Cinnamon rolls. There's a bakery in Santa Cruz that makes fabulous cinnamon rolls, almost as high as they are wide, and I think they put cinnamon in the dough, instead of just spreading a cinnamon sauce on plain dough before rolling it up.

Movie popcorn. I couldn't eat any when we saw *Ya-Ya Sisterhood*, and it smelled soooo good!

Oatmeal cookies. Homemade, with lots of raisins, fresh from the oven. I actually had a dream about them Friday morning.

Pastrami and Swiss on rye. Pastrami hot enough to melt the Swiss cheese, with lots of mustard and a dill pickle. And not that new lean stuff; I want the greasy, full-fat pastrami of my childhood! (That was Tuesday night's dream, shortly before the tongue transplant.)

Salad, almost any kind, but Chicken Caesar would be a nice start.

Pizza, almost any kind, but pepperoni has a special place in my heart.

Falafel from our favorite local restaurant.

And don't feel guilty if, after reading that list, your appetite gets a little over-stimulated and you go eat one of those items yourself. Enjoy it for me!

One-third done. Two weeks to replenish the supplies before Round Three, and after that round I'll be half-way there!

Loui

* * * * * * * * * * * * *

# SHORT AND SWEET

Sunday, July 21, 2002, 10:00 AM

This will be a short note because Sabine and I will be leaving soon to drive to an International Folk Dance Camp in Stockton, California (about an hour and half away). This year's curriculum includes dances from Bulgaria, Macedonia, Hungary, Turkey, Scandinavia, France, and the Pacific Islands. About 180 dancers come from all over the world to stay on the University of the Pacific campus for a week of learning new dances, dancing, talking about dances, dancing, thinking about dances, listening to dance music, dancing, listening to lectures about dance, dancing, eating while discussing the dances just taught, etc. We'll be back midday Sunday, July 28. While we're gone, the contractor who remodeled our kitchen and built our backyard gazebo is going to housesit for us and paint the interior of our townhouse! What a concept: we go away for a week and come home to a freshly painted house and don't have deal with the furniture moving, the mess, or the paint fumes!

This will also be the best week in my chemotherapy cycle, so I should have maximum energy, maximum red and white blood cells, maximum appetite.

The mouth problems that were plaguing me last week began clearing up Wednesday morning. Thank goodness, because five days of that was torture enough! Another day or two and I would have been rolling around on the floor, foaming at the mouth and babbling in an alien tongue. The Neupogen shots did the trick and my white blood cells came back in full force and began repairing the damage. The slime problem disappeared gradually, the sores healed, my taste buds are coming back, and my salivary glands now appear to be working again, though not with all the faucets fully open.

## GIGGLE OF THE WEEK

My giggle for the week came in the form of some photos from my friend Lee Myers. He saw one of the photographs taken by Bruce Meisner on my website and decided to have a little fun with it in Photoshop.

See the startling results at www.louitucker.com/MyersPhotos.htm

Round Three of chemotherapy starts Friday, July 26. Sabine and I will have to get up early, drive back to San Jose from Stockton for the treatments, and drive back for the afternoon dance classes. The doctor has promised he'll lower the dosages so I won't be so vulnerable to mouth problems (hallelujah!).

I hope you all enjoy your week as much as I'm going to enjoy mine!

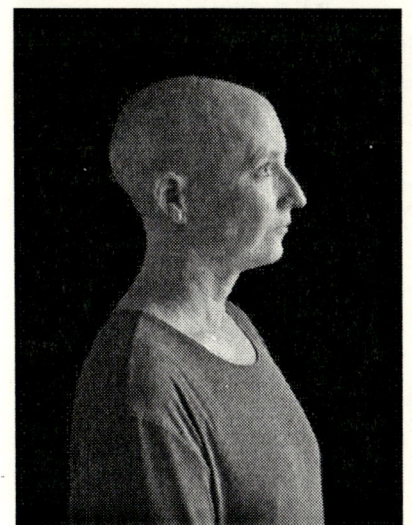 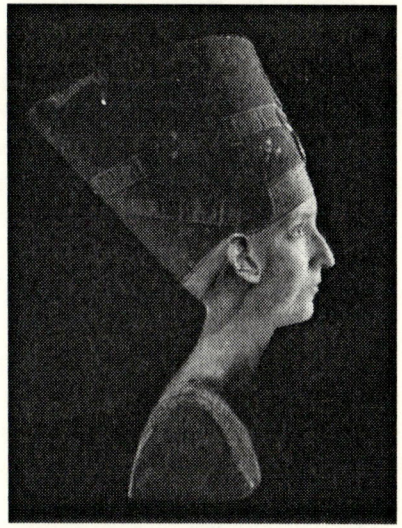

\* \* \* \* \* \* \* \* \* \* \* \* \* \*

# A CLOUD WITH A SILVER LINING

### Sunday, July 28, 2002, 8:00 PM

This past week was just about as wonderful as it could get given my medical challenges. I was fascinated to discover that saliva actually has a unique taste. You don't realize this until you don't have saliva for a while and it begins to come back. I could actually taste the change in my mouth! I had little welcome back celebrations for my taste buds every time I ate. A simple tomato sandwich (sourdough bread, mustard, mayo, thick slices of garden-fresh tomatoes) was so delicious it gave me goose bumps! Dinner Thursday night, in anticipation of chemo treatments starting the next morning, was sushi—YUUUMMMM! So from about Monday night on, I ate to my heart's content.

Friday morning, Sabine and I drove back to San Jose and showed up at the oncology clinic to begin Round Three. And I flunked my blood test! (If you could study for a blood test, I would have done so, instead of dancing until 1:30 AM!)

Clarification: I did in fact have blood. My red blood cell count was fine, but my white blood cell count was still too low to risk subjecting my system to chemotherapy. I had built up quite a supply of white blood cells with the Neupogen shots last week, but evidently most of those white blood cells were used up fixing the damage in my mouth. The white blood cell count wasn't zero again, just lower than was safe. The doctors felt it would be too risky to start Round Three because it would deplete my white blood cells even more and truly wipe out my immune system. An opportunistic infection wouldn't just make me uncomfortable, it would land me in the hospital. Lord knows I don't have time for that!

*Dancing with Cancer*

The bad news is that this means another week gets tacked on the end of my treatment, so some of the events I had scheduled in the future for "good" weeks are going to fall on "bad" weeks. I was warned by women who've had breast cancer treatment that this would probably happen, but I thought that I would stay strong and healthy and on track for the entire six months. Oh well.... If I flunk next month's blood test for the same reason, it will throw me off yet another week. Which reminds me of that saying: You wanna give God a good laugh? Make plans.

The silver lining in this otherwise gray cloud is that I have another entire week to eat whatever I want. I've gained back some of the weight I lost, but wouldn't mind putting a few more pounds back on. I have another week to enjoy the pretty-close-to-normal energy levels I've experienced this week. I will focus on these blessings.

So, can I anticipate suggestions from some of you reading this that I eat Substance X or drink Blah-de-Blah Tea or take XXX pills? Someone always seems to think ingesting something or other will help fix things. I've done some checking and I can't find anything definitive in the case of my white blood cells. There is all sorts of literature on the Internet and in bookstores about "blood tonics" but nothing specific or conclusive. Nobody has done a scientific study proving that if you take Substance X your white blood cell count will rise and if you don't take it the count will not rise. Why? Because your white blood cell count is going to go up anyway. That's just the way our bodies function. The oncology clinic staff has assured me that my body knows what it's doing and my white blood cell count will rise all by itself, without outside encouragement or intervention. The reason they gave me the Neupogen shots before was because I had NO white blood cells and I had a very obvious infection that required immediate attention. Right now I'm actually feeling fine, and I have no infections or other problems, so it is better to just let my body produce white blood cells as part of the natural process. If I want to drink some herbal concoction, I have been assured it will not hurt me, but why bother?

*Loui Tucker*

## THE MIRACLE OF THE HUMAN BODY

In the meantime, I confess that I am truly astonished at the human body's ability to take care of itself and do so efficiently and quietly. You probably don't notice, when you bruise yourself or cut yourself, how quickly the injury is repaired. I've recently experienced some pretty traumatic injuries, starting with two surgeries one week apart back in April, and two episodes of "mucousitis" (a.k.a. mouth sores). Once the healing starts, it is a daily miracle. I wake up each morning with a sense that restoration and reconstruction have taken place while I slept without causing so much as a hiccup. In contrast, when the roads, bridges, buildings and the like in our cities need repair, it cannot be done without roadblocks, detours, radio advisories, and general turmoil.

If you cut yourself and see some of your own blood, you probably don't give a second's thought to what a wondrous substance blood is. It's just a red liquid that hardens as it dries. Big deal. I now see my blood as containing fleets of tiny little cars and trucks and service vehicles whizzing along little highways in an interbody transit system that makes a mockery of our urban freeways. The red blood cells are the fully loaded trucks carrying supplies and equipment to organs and tissue. The white cells are the police and fire and ambulance services, the hazardous material squads, and the SWAT teams. I marvel at the fact that we humans have figured out where blood cells come from (who would imagine blood cell factories in our bone marrow?), how they mature, what they do, how long they live—especially given the fact that these cells cannot be seen with the naked eye!

## CHUCKLE OF THE WEEK

One of the dancers attending the camp this week walked up to me to share a story about a friend of hers who'd lost most of her hair during chemotherapy. She had soft peach fuzz all over her head.

Someone at a shopping mall came up to her and asked her where she got her hair done, that the style was exquisite and really suited her head. The woman smiled and, rather than go into a long explanation, simply wrote down the address of the hospital (without the name of the hospital) on a slip of paper, and suggested that the woman drop by and make an appointment....

## MY HERO

A good friend of mine also attended the same dance camp this week. She has been struggling with the after-effects of a variant of Guillain-Barr Syndrome which left her almost completely paralyzed 19 months ago (December 2000). A year ago, she was at dance camp, assisted by her husband. At that point, she could barely walk, could not feed or dress herself. She taught us a dance at a Recreational Dance Workshop while sitting in a chair and telling us what to do.

This year she was able to attend camp by herself, walking with a walker and a cane most of the time. She drives her own van with a handicapped placard. She can now dress and feed herself, but she struggles daily to build and retrain her muscles. She can grasp a fork and spoon, but cannot make a fist. Making a "thumbs up" sign is her current goal, since lifting her thumb requires some effort. In spite of all this, she participated in an "Experienced Square Dance" class each day. Don't pooh-pooh this on the grounds that square dancing is just walking. It's 45 minutes of non-stop, fast-paced walking, following directions, and working in tandem with seven other people in the square. She also attended most of the other dance classes and all the evening parties and shows. She was honored with an "Energizer Bunny" award for her keep-on-truckin'-never-say-die-I-just-gotta-dance attitude. When you realize what she's had to overcome, and she's done it with grace and a smile on her face and a ready laugh—it's hard to complain about a few aches and pains and a little one-year setback like breast cancer and chemotherapy and being bald for a few months. She's been fighting her way back for 18 months! Linda, you are my hero!

Loui Tucker

Count your blessings and give thanks for your good health, folks. Wishing you a good week,

              Loui

* * * * * * * * * * * * *

# ROUND THREE OF SIX BEGINS

### Sunday August 4, 2002, 7:30 PM

So I'm back on track again. All week I ate and worked and danced and slept like the pre-April, 2002 Loui. I had a grand ol' time!

Friday my blood showed I was healthy enough to withstand the onslaught of another round of chemotherapy, so here I am. Round Three, Part One is hard at work in me as I write. My doctor reduced the drug dosages a bit to try to avoid the worst of the mouth problems. I'm also stopping the oral medication two days early and getting a variant of Neupogen to attempt to get my white blood cells counts back up more efficiently.

At least this time, I know pretty much what to expect. I'll have a dry mouth, little or no saliva, and toasted taste buds, but nothing I haven't dealt with before. No surprises and, if I'm lucky, no sores and no slime (please!).

**NIGHT SWEATS**

It was not actually a surprise, but this side effect started recently for me. You may already know that chemotherapy induces menopause. Footnote: for women who get breast cancer in their 30s or earlier, their periods often resume after the chemo is over, much like their hair grows back. There are many examples of women who have children AFTER going through chemotherapy for cancer.

Anyway, I've started with night sweats. Call me crazy if you like, but I am actually enjoying them at times. No, really—I am!

Remember what it's like on a really hot muggy August day when you're just melting with the heat and you dive into a pool of cool water. Remember how shocking and wonderful it feels? Well, night sweats remind me of that experience.

First, you wake up feeling overheated. You push down the blankets a little, then push them farther down, finally throw them all the way to the end of the bed. Your exposed skin (the more the better—sleep in the nude if you can) is suddenly in contact with lots of cold air. If a window near the bed is left open, it's even better. You get that same delicious, almost giggle-producing wave of pleasure from the relief and release of the heat. It feels like there is steam rising from your body. A minute later, you're cool and comfortable and you reach to pull the sheets up around you. Turn over, and you're back to sleep (at least I am.) Total elapsed time: maybe two minutes. I'll grant you it's annoying when it happens every two hours or so all night, but at least the interruptions are brief.

## VALIDATION

This week I got some validation in the "writing as therapy" department. Cliff shared with me an article he found called "Writing Your Wrongs." I don't know the source. I won't re-print the entire article but here's the gist of it:

> "…the act of writing is good not only for your mind, but for your immune system as well…. James Pennebacker of the University of Texas at Austin and Joshua Smith of Syracuse University have found that people facing life-threatening illnesses can boost their immune function if they write about their emotions and stress."

The two researchers worked with HIV/AIDS patients, and asked one group to write about their daily schedule and another group to write about negative life experiences.

> "Those who dipped into the inkwell of life experience showed a quantifiable increase in immune functioning. The researchers found that the mere expression of emotions on paper isn't enough to boost health—the writer must apply focused thought and use the words to actually interpret his or her experience."

Who knew???

## BALDNESS AS A TEACHING TOOL

There is, in the breast cancer school of thought, an adage that goes something like this: If you behave as if you feel well, you WILL FEEL well. If you put on a smile, you WILL FEEL like smiling. If you laugh, you WILL FEEL the humor. Breast cancer patients are encouraged to wear a wig, put on makeup, dress for the day and put on an outward appearance that says everything is just hunky-dory. Doctors will write prescriptions for wigs so that insurance will cover the cost. There are entire businesses devoted to selling scarves and other headwear for women whose hair has thinned or disappeared completely. Women wear false eyelashes and carefully paint on eyebrows. And don't forget the reconstruction surgery and prosthesis business for women who have had mastectomies.

Women do all this for a variety of reasons: (1) to maintain a sense of normalcy for the sake of children; (2) personal vanity; (3) to preserve desirability in an intimate relationship; even (4) fear of discrimination at work (getting passed over for a long-term project if it is felt that you'll be too ill to handle it).

So I walk around bald pretty much 22/7. I'm guessing it's not 24/7, since I often have to deal with chilly offices and restaurants and carry a scarf that I can quickly wrap around my head. To deal with the four reasons mentioned above: (1) I have no children who need a sense of normalcy, (2) I like to look good, but I've never been particularly vain; (3) Sabine thinks my baldness is adorable; and (4) I've been an independent contractor for almost 20 years and have little fear of losing clients or jobs. If anything, I'm the one cutting back so I can rest in the afternoons. You can add to that the fact that even the THOUGHT of dancing aerobically for two or three hours at a stretch in a wig makes me break out in a sweat!

I think another reason I choose to be bald in public (other than comfort) is that I am, at my core, a teacher. I have been a teacher most of my adult life. I taught in the California public schools for eight years. After that I worked for a company that sold dedicated word processors (back before computers had software such as WordPerfect, WordStar and Word) and taught recent purchasers how to use their new equipment. In my current business, part of my work is training people how to use their computer software more productively. Most of you know that I've taught dance classes for over 20 years.

Being publicly bald is like being a life-sized teaching aid. I get into conversations with parking lot attendants, restaurant staff, receptionists, and grocery store clerks. "Hey, cool summer hairdo" is how it usually starts. I respond with something like, "Well, it's not entirely voluntary. I'm receiving chemotherapy for breast cancer and a side effect is that I've lost all my hair." I tell them survival rates are very high for breast cancer, that I'm not in any grave danger, or contagious, and that I'm feeling fine considering the chemicals floating around in my bloodstream.

At some point I advise the (female) listener to either get regular mammograms or (male listeners) make sure their female loved ones get them. I remind them that early detection can mean the difference between Stage One cancer and Stage Four cancer (I have Stage Two). I hope it also means that some of these people will not toss in the trash that unsolicited mail from the American Cancer Society or the Breast Cancer Research Fund and decide instead to mail a check because they saw and talked to me.

I'm not suggesting that every woman who has to go through cancer treatment should do it my way, or that if they choose to wear a wig they are somehow a wimp, afraid of how they'll be treated. This is my way. Every woman, every body is different. We have different life situations and schlep different emotional baggage around with us. We react to the chemicals differently, and we react to the stress differently. For some women, nausea is a big deal, but they never get mouth sores. I'm the other way around. I just find that being a teacher and staying a teacher gives a purpose to the process.

Just think, this time NEXT week, I'll be almost half way through!

Loui

* * * * * * * * * * * * *

# TWO MORE DAYS AND I'M HALF WAY!

### August 11, 2002, 8:30 PM

This Tuesday I take the last of the oral medication for Round Three. I'll have to stop by the oncology clinic to get a white blood cell booster this Friday and have a stress test next Friday but, for all intents and purposes, I'm just two days away from being half way through the chemotherapy treatment.

What does half way mean exactly? I had been thinking of it as reaching the top of a hill, knowing it's just downhill from here. That's not the case according to most cancer treatment staff. The second half is harder than the first half even though they may lower the dosage. Your body and blood just don't recover completely during the time off so you go into each Round a little depleted. Despite that, I'm still going to think of this as getting to the top of the hill and looking at the downhill section. It may not be *physically* easier, but it will *psychologically* be easier.

It's not just three drinks gone out of a six pack, or five kilometers finished in a 10K run, or 4½ months passing in a pregnancy. It's like Wednesday lunch during a workweek. Sure, the deadline is still looming on Friday and the hours will become longer and the work will undoubtedly get more stressful, but it's just 2.5 days until the weekend—and downhill is still downhill.

On Wednesday I'm going to change the belt on my "Karate Teddy Bear" from The Vermont Teddy Bear Company. I got this cute-as-a-bug gift from Lynn. (To read more about them, go to www.vermontteddybear.com—a great alternative to sending flowers!) It's a teddy bear in a karate outfit (with "Loui" emblazoned on the back!) and comes with a set of six belts—black, white, red, green, yellow, and blue. As I complete each Round, I am going to celebrate by changing the bear's belt. Around the middle of November, I'll have a black belt in cancer fighting! (To tell the truth, I don't think of this as cancer fighting. The drugs are doing all the fighting, not me! I just have to survive the side effects that the drugs cause!)

When I look at what I've written the last two times I've gotten to this point in the cycle, it's been about dry mouth and mouth sores. It has not been quite so bad this time. I've got that lump in my throat that makes it difficult to swallow, and my saliva is down by at least half, so I'm back to liquids and soft, moist food. My taste buds are mostly gone except for the ones that process fructose (fruit sugar), so fruit is still nice to eat. Somehow it just does not seem as bad as before. Maybe it's because I haven't felt or seen any real mouth sores or fungus (yet?). Maybe it's because, by now, this is a familiar sort of discomfort, one I know how to handle, one I know will be gone in a week or so. Either way, I'm coping better. Saturday night and Sunday are still my lowest times, from an energy standpoint, but I expect to be working and dancing by tomorrow.

## MAMMOGRAMS AND SELF-EXAMS

I wrote a couple of weeks ago about the importance of mammograms. I didn't mention, and should have mentioned, the importance of frequent breast self-exams for women (men, your job is to tell your female loved ones about this). Some of the women I talked with about this have said things like, "My breast are naturally lumpy. How am I going to feel anything unusual?" or "I have all these cysts and crystallized patches. I'll never be able to feel if anything is growing." As if these were excuses that would relieve you of the job!

Look at it this way: sure, it's easy to find weeds in a back yard that is 99% open grass because the weeds stand out clearly. If you have a back yard that's got flowering shrubs and trees and a vegetable patch along with the grass, you've just got to learn the landscape and be vigilant and aware. If you're familiar with what's supposed to be there, you're sure to spot a foreign growth in your strawberry patch (so to speak).

## FORWARDING E-MAIL

By the way, it's perfectly okay to forward these e-mails to friends and relatives. You don't have to ask permission. This certainly cannot be considered private e-mail when it's going out to over 200 people already! If you prefer, just send me the addresses and I'll add them to my list.

## MY FAVORITE PHOTOGRAPHER

One last thing: A few local readers have asked for more details about Bruce Meisner, the man who took the professional photographs of me and Sabine. Check out his website at www.bmeisner.com. You'll see more samples of his work, read about his focus and style, and be able to contact him directly.

## ANECDOTE

A man goes into a health club for his twice weekly session with his personal trainer. While waiting for the trainer to arrive, his routine is to warm up on the treadmill. He isn't careful and happens to step onto a treadmill that was left running. Of course, he goes up in the air and down on the floor, banging and scraping knees and shins. The staff ministers to him, applying disinfectant and salves and bandages. The personal trainer arrives, looks at his miserable client, who is longing for some quiet time on a bed with some ice packs. The personal trainer smiles and says, "Okay, today we'll just do upper body work."

There is a lesson there somewhere, but I'm not sure I'm ready to write about it…..

## WORDS I WANT TO LIVE BY

People will forget what you said, people will forget what you did, but people will never forget how you made them feel. (Carl W. Buechner)

Enjoy your week, your work, your friends. And rejoice: you too must be half way to somewhere!

Loui

* * * * * * * * * * * * *

## A 4 ON A SCALE OF 1-10

### August 18, 2002, 9:30 PM

I go to sleep with a combination meditation/visualization to ease me into sleep and encourage my body to rebuild. The past few nights have been this one:

I imagine a microscopic manager with a teensy-weensy clipboard, preparing the troops for night action.

"Okay, listen up! We've gotten some reinforcements, but there's a lot of work to be done. There's still the digestive tracts to clear out, so the regular crews will be working there. You might as well get going. Rich and David, you take Units 85–98 and deal with the cat scratches on her left hand. Lynn and Chris, you take Units 99–112 and start in on the paper cuts on her right hand and if you get done there before daybreak, she's got some blisters on her right foot.

"Maude and Ralph, I know you are getting tired of this particular duty, but we need you back in her mouth. Don't give me that look! You two are the veterans and you know what you're up against. This is not a job for amateurs. There's a fire pit in the back left corner of her tongue, her gums are tender, and I've gotten numerous reports that the top of her throat has something going on that's impeding the passage of food. Take Units 113–200 and do what you can. It may take a couple of shifts. And I promise, and I mean it this time, I *promise* you at least 10 days R&R, and I'm working on getting you a trip to the beach and all the piña coladas you drink. Okay, that's it, everybody get going!"

So far it has not worked. (Sigh!) I remain hopeful, of course, that tonight will be the night. I'll run the show once again and in the morning I'll have a new mouth....

## FOOD IS NOT FUN....YET!

This Round Three has not been as bad as prior months. If last month, with the multiple sores, the tongue replacement, and slime was about a 12 on a scale of 1 to 10, this month was about a 4. I've been able to eat so I have not lost any more weight. Not a sore mouth really, just tender except for the one bad spot.

Most meals involve one of those four-way meetings between my nose, my eyes, my stomach, and my brain. Food continues to smell wonderful (popcorn, fresh bread, pizza, take-out from the local barbecue joint...). In fact, Friday night I sat for several minutes and held a cube of fresh whole wheat challah under my nose and just enjoyed the smell of it. I knew I'd be crazy to try to eat it, but the aroma was fabulous! Of course, my eyes still work and food looks just fine. My stomach is usually on red alert, ready for any deliveries. It's my brain (a.k.a. Pain Central) that's got this checklist:

(1) is it liquid?
(2) is it soft?
(3) is it spicy, salty, crisp, crunchy, or dry?
(4) will it require a lot of chewing and saliva?
(5) do you *promise* to take very small bites and chew it *really well*?

Sometimes, I eat it anyway and suffer. Sometimes my taste buds, which just this weekend started making a reappearance, report that the nose overplayed it a bit because the food didn't taste as good as it smelled. So I can eat. I'm just cautious. And I confess, I am getting really tired of soup! I can promise you this: as soon as Maude and Ralph do their thing in my mouth, I'm going to be putting in some serious time at the dining room table!

## 8 OUT OF 9

Eight out of nine *what,* you ask? Well, the statistic that gets bandied about is "1 out of 9 women will face breast cancer in her lifetime." It's the most common form of cancer in women in the U.S. and there are almost 160,000 cases diagnosed each year in the U.S. (See all the good company I've got!)

"1 out of 9" sells mammograms. "1 out of 9" sells thousands of those little plastic signs to hang in showers that promote breast self-exams. "1 out of 9" is supposed to chill you into changing your eating habits, your stress-level, your exercise routine, even your residence. Well, "1 out of 9" also turns women into hypochondriacs! It's the same as saying not only is the glass half empty, but there is a hole in the bottom!

Not that I'm discounting any of that. After all, I am one of those nine and it has not been fun. Women really should get mammograms and do breast self-exams, especially after age 40. However, I find a great deal of reassurance in thinking "8 out of 9 women WILL NOT get breast cancer!" I nagged Sabine until she got her mammogram done (she's turning 40 this year—October 19 in case anyone wants to write that down) and we were relieved when the report came back that she's clear. I am comforted by the thought that she's safe, at least for now. Maybe it's the cockeyed optimist in me, but "8 out of 9" sounds very comforting right now.

You know what puts women at a high risk for breast cancer? Well, it's not diet, number of pregnancies, fertility or birth control drugs, exercise, exposure to pesticides, alcohol consumption, hormone replacement therapy for menopause, or even ethnicity. It's not so easy to say, "This causes breast cancer, so don't do it." In fact, I have read that if you look at the list of various factors that contribute to your risk of getting breast cancer, 70% of breast cancer patients have none of the classical risk factors. While I was not in that 70% group, I had three risk factors—I am over age 50, I took birth control pills, and I have had no pregnancies. And in case you were wondering, I had not taken hormone replacement therapy.

All the things I listed above are factors, for sure, but number one on the list is: a blood relative who has had breast cancer. Imagine the surprise for my sister and my nieces when they are told they are now at a higher risk for breast cancer because I had breast cancer. Nothing about their lives has changed, but my diagnosis means they are now SIX TIMES more at risk! It's a crazy world, isn't it?

## R&R

So this week and next week will be R&R. Rest, recovery, recuperation, rebuilding, and recreation. And eating. No drugs and no pain (assuming Maude and Ralph get busy later tonight while I'm asleep) for almost two weeks. It will be my longest pain-free-drug-free period since mid-April when this all got started with the two surgeries (biopsy, then lumpectomy & lymphedectomy). Wow! Go head, ask me if I'm excited about this! (You betcha, by golly, I sure am!)

## WAY TO LOOK AT IT

"Life is like a tea bag. It's only when we're put in hot water that we find out how strong we are." (I'm not sure who said it first, but I read it in a book by Rita Mae Brown.)

*Loui Tucker*

When you sit down to eat a good meal this week, imagine me eating one too!

Loui

* * * * * * * * * * * * *

# GETTING GRUMPY

## August 25, 2002, 9:30 PM

I've tried to keep smiling, or at least maintain a stiff upper lip, about all that is happening to me, but this weekend, I have to report a flaming case of the Grumpies.

First, the night sweats are contributing to my fatigue. It is bad enough that my blood chemistry limits me in the energy department, but I can't get a full night's sleep, and that makes me even groggier in the afternoon. You may remember from a past e-mail that chemotherapy dumps female recipients into menopause (it blocks the output of estrogen). This by itself has not been a major inconvenience. I've had a few mild hot flashes during the day but none of the wild mood swings associated with menopause (at least not yet).

Even the night sweats by themselves are not a big deal—a two- or three-minute interruption. The problem is the frequency; they happen about every two hours. You know the nights (or early mornings) when you fall into bed, turn over once and you're out like a light, and then you wake up 6 or 7 or 8 hours later in the same position? That's what I call "dead to the world, like a moss-covered log in dreamless darkness, bone-quenching, soul-healing" sleep. That is the kind of sleep I can't get, and have not gotten for about a month now. I sleep in two-hour chunks, and deep, dreamless sleep eludes me. Eight hours *in bed* feels very different from eight hours of *sleep*.

Couple the night sweats with the lowered red blood cells, and napping in the afternoon is becoming not just advisable, if I want to do anything in the evening, but a requirement. Which is what is annoying me. The hour or two taken out of each afternoon is cutting into my time for walking and reading and doing paperwork and returning phone calls and—whatever I want to do. It is interfering with my life! If there is a solution or remedy, other than to lie back, take that nap, and accept it as a temporary fact of my life, I don't know what it is.

My other annoyance is more cosmetic and I know I'll get accustomed to it with time, but right now it's making me grumpy. I had counted myself as lucky because I had not lost my eyelashes and eyebrows. As it turned out, I was not actually lucky, just behind schedule. My eyelashes and eyebrows had been getting increasingly thinner over the last month, and this week the last of the lashes finally gave up and left. My eyebrows are down to about eight individual hairs each, and I don't imagine they will last through the end of the month.

I know I will get used to the way it looks, just as I got used to looking in mirrors and seeing myself bald, but at the moment it bothers me that I look so alien. I suppose I will experiment with eyeliners and eyebrow pencils, which may help my outlook but, in the meantime, this latest turn in the long dark tunnel is not making me happy! I wish I could find some solace in knowing I'm saving several hundred dollars over the course of the cancer treatment not paying for haircuts, hair products, and makeup. Sigh!

## MY NEW RESPONSE

The next time someone makes a comment about being bald, and tells me, "Oh, but you have such a nice shaped head!" I'm going to respond: "Thanks! I'm been working out. All those hours in the gym are finally paying off. Great muscle tone, huh?" (Sorry, more grumpiness....)

## FOOD, GLORIOUS FOOD!

On the positive front, meals were delightful events this week. My saliva and taste buds came back gradually, as I expected, and by Thursday I had a normal-feeling mouth. The process reminds me of a film I saw in some science class eons ago, which showed a tide pool over a 12-hour period, using time-lapse photography. It started with the tide pool looking lush and hydrated, full of sea life and plants waving about in the water. The tide receded, and you could watch the animals burrow into the sand and hide under rocks and in crevasses. The plants turned into lumps of glop, like damp laundry on the rocks and sand. The tide came back, the animals came out of hiding, the plant life plumped up and everything was back to the way it was at the beginning of the film clip. That pretty much describes the monthly cycle of my mouth!

## KNOW YOUR SIDE EFFECTS

There are two schools of thought when it come to telling patients about side effects. One schools runs with the "ignorance is bliss" theory. You should limit what patients know about side effects of the medicines they are taking because knowing about them may increase fear and anxiety about taking the medication in the first place, and may actually cause some suggestible patients to imagine or even generate the side effects (Ah, the power of the mind!).

The other school of thought holds to the "knowledge is power" and "what you don't know can hurt you" theories. My doctors belong to this group and, after last week, I'm very glad.

One of the side effects of the medication I'm taking to encourage the manufacture of white blood cells is what they call bone pain. I was told to expect an aching in my large bones (my pelvis, thighs, sternum, etc.), depending on where the medication settled. The first month the sensation was in my pelvis: "WHUMP, WHUMp, WHUmp, Whump, Whump, whump, whmp, whm...." It's a sort of throbbing that fades away in about ten beats. The first time it hits it is quite startling ("What was THAT????") and I can imagine being really panicked if I hadn't been told to expect it. The throbbing happens intermittently every couple of hours or so for several days. I've now come to welcome the throbbing as a sign that my WBC are coming back and any sores I have will soon be gone.

Now, imagine when those throbbing sensations suddenly happen in your breastbone and sternum, which is where they occurred this month for me! If I had not been prepared, I'd have been in the car heading for the emergency room, frantic that I was having a heart attack! The lesson I learned: know ALL the possible side effects of the medication you are taking. Forewarned is forearmed.

## ROUND FOUR COMING UP

Assuming my white blood cells are ready for the onslaught, I start Round Four this Friday. Sabine and I hope to enjoy Friday and Saturday in the Santa Cruz Mountains courtesy of Cliff and Terry before I head for the covers for the expected downtime next Sunday.

Three months gone, three months to go. Looking backward, the LAST three months seem to have gone quickly, but looking ahead, the NEXT three months is the same length of time but seems like SUCH a long haul ahead! I try to stay focused on Thanksgiving, when all this chemotherapy will be over and my taste buds will be getting ready for sweet potatoes, cranberry sauce, and pumpkin pie.

So, my wide circle of friends and supporters, send those strengthening, encouraging waves my way. This month I'm feeling more in need of them than before.

Loui

\* \* \* \* \* \* \* \* \* \* \* \* \*

# OKAY, SO I'M HUMAN TOO!

## Sunday, September 1, 2002, 9:30 PM

Judging from some of the e-mail responses I got last week, I think I may have overstated my case. I wrote that I was grumpy, just *GRUMPY*—not disabled, not distraught, not depressed, not ready to throw in the towel, for heaven's sake! Some of you readers seemed to think I was stopping all my work and my dancing in order to spend all my time napping. Perish the thought! I was in a funk for a couple of days, but I got over it.

Some of my ability to crawl out of that emotional hole was thanks to some well-pointed e-mail from y'all. To paraphrase a few of them:

**GLAD YOU'RE ONE OF US**: "It's about time you started showing signs of being human. All that cheerful, strong, good-humored, I-sure-am-a-tough-old-bird posturing was only good for so long, you know. Glad to see you too can get the blues."

**GET REAL #1**: "So you don't get a full night's sleep! Welcome to the world of families with newborns. Newborns need to be fed about every two hours (and wake you up noisily to tell you about it) and that's for the first 10–12 weeks of their little lives! Just remember it doesn't last forever."

**GET REAL #2**: "So you get tired! So you have to take a nap! Be glad you have a work situation that allows you to set your own hours and take a nap if you want to, because otherwise you'd be working full time and toughing it out, or working part time, or on disability, or taking a leave of absence. Be glad taking a nap because you're tired is the extent of your limitations, because you could be waiting for a kidney transplant and submitting yourself to four hours of dialysis three days a week. Let's get a little perspective here."

**GLAMOUR ISN'T EVERYTHING**: "I know someone who lost her eyebrows during chemotherapy and got so used to the way she looked without them that, when they grew back in, she felt her 'new' eyebrows were too thick and bushy and made her look like Groucho Marx!"

**YOU'RE IN GOOD COMPANY**: "I haven't checked to be sure, but I've been told Mona Lisa didn't have eyebrows either!"

**THE BENCHMARK WAS TOO HIGH ANYWAY**: "I was beginning to worry that if I showed your e-mails to future breast cancer patients that they'd feel they too would be expected to show your level of energy, good spirits, and savvy. The last e-mail you sent cut them some slack!"

So I am coping with the night sweats and the alien-looking eyes. To answer a few other questions, sleeping pills are not an option. I don't have trouble *falling* asleep or *getting back* to sleep. The problem is being awakened every two hours by a body that's running a fever, steaming, and begging for release from the sheets. I have tried to imagine what would happen if I was so drugged by a sleeping aid that I did not wake up. I don't know whether I'd implode or explode, melt or vaporize.

The night sweats are brought on by estrogen depletion and deprivation. The cancer drugs block the production of estrogen because estrogen contributes to tumor growth in the type of cancer I have. Taking estrogen or estrogen-like substitutes is considered either counterproductive or futile. It is assumed the cancer drugs will negate any possible benefit. HRT and other hormone (estrogen) replacement therapies are not advisable on chemo. There are reports of a few brave souls who are taking HRT despite the risks and advice against it, because they cannot manage the hot flashes and prefer to take their chances, but it is too early to tell if there will be any long-lasting consequences.

As for the missing eyebrows and eyelashes—oh, well. A little makeup helps, but it's a look I will get used to, just as I got used to being bald.

## ROUND FOUR, WEEK ONE

So Friday morning of this past week I started Round Four and, as usual, I felt fine and had plenty of energy and appetite for about 36 hours. Sabine and I spent the night at Cliff and Terry's place in the Santa Cruz Mountains, along with about 30 other campers. Treats: dinner cooked over and eaten around a campfire, watching the kids toast marshmallows and make S'mores, dancing on that huge deck under the trees, meeting and greeting old friends. More of the same the next day. I started to fade in the late afternoon, so we drove home and by 5:30 PM I was down for the count. Sundays! Will I ever get used to that dragged-down, listless, beyond simply tired, washed-out feeling on the Sundays after chemo? All I want to do is sleep, which is about all I do, except for getting up every couple of hours to deal with the sweats. I got up for a light meal about 10:30 AM and went right back to bed.

By Sunday evening, I'm able to sit and read e-mail, write this piece, pay some bills and do other paperwork, but that's about it. If past months are any indication, I'll be pretty much recovered from the Sunday Slump by tomorrow morning. It's just one really low day at a time, two Sundays per month. I know cancer patients who have to live with much worse.

## GRATEFUL FOR COBRA

My medical bills have, for the most part, been covered by my husband's (yes, we're still married) medical coverage. John turns 65 this September and he will be shifted from that medical plan to MediCal. In order to continue my coverage under that old plan, I will have to pay the monthly fees under COBRA. I always thought COBRA stood for something like "Continuation of Benefits Reassurance Act" or at least something descriptive of what the federal legislation (1986, by the way) was designed to do. Hah! COBRA stands for "Consolidated Omnibus Budget Reconciliation

Act." In the event that ever comes up on a trivia quiz or in a crossword puzzle, you'll know.

Anyway, the COBRA payment to continue my medical coverage for myself is $400+ per month—whew! It seems like a lot, but it sure beats paying the weekly bills from the oncology clinic and the prescriptions! I looked at the charges and *each* chemo treatment is over $700 and I get two per month, which does not include the miscellaneous blood tests, and shots of Neupogen, etc. Changing insurance coverage at this point is just about impossible. What company will accept a cancer patient? I'll have to wait until this is all over and then look for a cheaper alternative. Maybe by then Sabine will have domestic partner benefits through her school district and I can get coverage through her?

## THERE ARE BOOKS, AND THERE ARE BOOKS

I have gotten so many gifts in the past months. I have not, could not, acknowledge them all. Besides the shoebox stuffed full of cards, I have received a dozen hats, scarves, and miscellaneous head coverings, CDs of soothing music, fans, posters and wall-hangings, scented candles, food (!), and books, books, books. (Whine: If I didn't have to *WASTE* so much valuable time *NAPPING*, I might actually get to *READ* some of the books.) I have received books about cancer, books written by and about cancer survivors, and books on other subjects to help me take my mind off cancer.

One tip for gift-givers, especially when it comes to books: Check the copyright date. If it's about coping with cancer treatment and its side effects, the book should not be more than two years old. So much happens so quickly in cancer treatment that a book that is five years old or more will probably give the reader an inaccurate picture of what is involved. For example, I was certain I would be dealing with massive nausea but, because of the advancements in treating that particular side effect, that has been the least of my worries.

The very best book you can buy a breast cancer patient is *Dr. Susan Love's Breast Book*. (Aside: when I first heard the title, I thought it was by someone named Dr. Susan who loves breasts.) It's thick and heavy, but it's a terrific resource. Dr. Love has been working in the field of breast cancer research for decades and her book is now in its third edition. It's about as up to date and accurate a book on breast cancer as you are going to find. In fact, if you're worried about breast cancer, get it now and read it, particularly the chapters about risks and prevention.

DO NOT GIVE A BREAST CANCER PATIENT EITHER *What Your Doctor Will Not Tell You About Breast Cancer* or *Love, Medicine & Miracles*. The first of the two books points, erroneously, to drugs and bad diets that are believed to cause breast cancer. While all of the points made are valid, they are only valid to the extent they are risk factors. None of the items mentioned in this book (birth control pills, HRT, etc.) directly *CAUSE* breast cancer.

The second book contains some good messages that promote positive thinking in the form of meditation, hypnotherapy, visualization, etc. as aids in healing. Fine, I subscribe to all that. Unfortunately the author takes a big leap beyond healing to causation (these are actual quotes from the book!):

> "The simple truth is, happy people generally don't get sick." (page 76)

> "My own father developed lung cancer shortly after retiring. At first it was hard for him to admit the significance of his retirement. Fortunately, after surgery, he was able to find fulfillment in his life, and the disease has not recurred in over twelve years." (page 81)

> "As a woman who developed cancer after her children left home expressed it in a letter to me, 'I had an empty

place in me, and the cancer grew to fill it.'" (page 81)
"The truth is that compulsively proper and generous people predominate among cancer patients because they put the needs of others ahead of their own. Cancer might be called the disease of nice people." (page 94)

"…those who develop cancer have often felt a sense of despair about their lives for months or years…." (page 102)

Oh really? Besides defying medical reality (most cancers take many years to grow and aren't going to pop up overnight in response to life situations), the author seems to take delight in blaming people for getting a disease. "You got this because you don't love yourself enough." "In your deepest psyche you needed this disease." Yikes!

What earthly good does it do to tell people who are fighting a disease, whether it's cancer or something else, that they are sick through some failure on their part? Even if your friend actually causes a bad accident, is re-living the accident over and over to understand what he or she did wrong going to help the healing process? The curative powers of guilt—what a belief system!

Besides, from every bit of reading I've done, there are no known, for-sure, slam-dunk absolute "causes" of cancer. Yes, the risk of getting lung cancer if you smoke is dramatic, but there are plenty of examples of people who smoked (or were exposed to asbestos) for decades and never got lung cancer. There are hundreds of thousands of people who exhibit major risk factors—obesity, alcohol consumption, drug abuse, fatty diet, little exercise, high stress, family history of cancer, and so on—and they don't get cancer, and yet there are health-conscious marathon runners and personal trainers who do.

Add to that the fact that there are lots of risk factors over which you have no control. For example, one of the charts in *Dr. Susan Love's Breast Book* shows the relative risks for different ethnic groups: White women are at the highest risk, then Black women, then Hispanic women, then Asian women. (An interesting footnote: when Asian women come to the U.S., their risk of breast cancer goes up.)

Even stress by itself is not a risk factor; it's how you *react* to stress that creates the risk. Do you bottle up all that stress, eat junk food, sleep poorly, and veg out mindlessly in front of the television? Or do you take time to write or talk about your problems that are causing the stress, eat well, get enough sleep, and exercise?

All the research and studies indicate there seems to be a genetic pre-disposition and a whole lot of risk factors or triggers. After that, getting cancer is about as much your fault as getting hit by a car while crossing a street to buy lunch. Sure, you could have chosen a different place for lunch, or you could have eaten at your desk, thus avoiding crossing the street, but getting hit by that car is still not your fault.

Okay, I've gone on long enough, way more than recently, but I needed to get a lot out this week. Considering how exhausted I felt all day, I'm feeling pretty pumped up right now. Those books in particular were taking up a lot of psychic space, weighing me down, and writing about them helped clear that out of my system. Ironically, the people who gave me the two books do not even have computers or e-mail, so they will not even see what I have written!

I did a little re-calculation this month. Instead of thinking in terms of chemo treatments (this one plus five more) or even months (two and a half), I'm going to count weeks: 10 weeks to go. Count down: 10, 9, 8, 7, .... That seems pretty easy. Just 10 weeks and I'll be done with all the pills and chemicals. Then two weeks to recover and four weeks of radiation. Piece of cake! I can do this.

All my thanks for your support and good wishes.

Loui

* * * * * * * * * * * * *

# THOUGHTS AFTER ANOTHER SLOW SUNDAY

September 8, 2002, 8:30 PM

Except for this being one of my typical weak-as-a-newborn-kitten Sundays, I'm fine. The Adriamycin chemotherapy (also known as the Red Devil because it's about the color of cherry Jell-O on Friday wiped me out again, so I slept most of today. My throat feels like the sores there have opened up again, but other than that, I'm fine. It was another of those "4 on a scale of 1–10" weeks. This coming week I'll be back to my liquid-soft-bland diet, but at least I know what to expect and what I can and cannot do.

There is something pitifully reassuring about a familiar pain, a been-here-done-this kind of pain. It's not a whoa-what-is-happening-to-me-now-do-I-need-to-call-the-doctor kind of pain. I'll finish the oral medication on Tuesday, have a white-blood-cell booster on Wednesday, and then I'm off-duty until Sept. 27 when I start Round Five.

As I knew I would, I'm getting used to the lack of eyebrows and eyelashes. I'm getting pretty good at drawing on eyebrows and lining my eyes. Sure, they look drawn on from up close, but at least I don't frighten the folks standing in line at the grocery store.

My weight is holding steady. I haven't been able to gain back any of the weight I've lost, but I have stopped losing, which is a good thing. I've already had my dress pants taken in and I've bought several new pairs of jeans. I don't want to repeat the process again in two months.

## INADVERTENT WISDOM

I have a number of young (under age 13) dancers in my Monday dance class. One of them came up to me a couple of weeks ago, after I sent out the e-mail about being half way through my cancer treatments, and said, "My father told me that you are half way through your testing and I'm glad. I hope you pass your tests and you never have to do this again."

Tests? Hmm.... Why "tests?" I recently asked the father (who is also a dancer in my class) about this choice of words. The family language is Hebrew so of course the father had talked about my health situation with his family in Hebrew. He explained to me that he'd used the word "tipulim" for "treatments." Evidently that was not a familiar word so "tests" became the reasonable guess. After all, you go to doctors when you are sick and doctors give you the results after you take tests, and then you get better. It was absolutely logical.

My young dancer's goal was communication and communication was accomplished. I got the message that I was cared about, and that my progress and health were being watched. I think now that the choice of words was inadvertently very wise because the word "testing" stuck with me for several days and I told several people about that conversation. It opened a door into a room in my mind that I had not thought to enter. We all get tested in life, in our jobs, and in our relationships. We get tested physically, mentally, spiritually, and emotionally. Having cancer and experiencing cancer treatment is a major life test, like the SAT and GMAT, the tests that decide the course of our careers and in some ways our lives. Beyond being a test of your body's tolerance for some wickedly powerful chemicals, cancer and cancer treatment are tests of your strength and stamina, your wit and will, even your character. This cancer test is definitely changing my outlook and attitudes toward people and life; I expect that when it is all over it will have altered more than that.

*Loui Tucker*

## TREATS THIS WEEK

I have been accused of being entirely too optimistic, light-hearted, and positive for my own reality. You know the expression about seeing the world through rose-colored glasses? Well, that's me. It hasn't always been this way. I did some therapy in my mid-30s and rid myself of chronic depression, along with some heavy emotional baggage and inner turmoil, and that resulted in most of this up-beat attitude of mine.

And now I am the proud owner of a pair of rose-colored glasses, courtesy of a thoughtful friend. Thank you, Ann!

## NIGHT SWEATS

I got a commiserating e-mail from a woman who used to dance in my Thursday dance class (she moved out of the area a few years ago and we MISS HER!) all about night sweats and hot flashes and the various joys of menopause. It was the subject line of her e-mail that had me in giggles: From a fellow "night sweater." The image that came instantly to mind was of a light weight cardigan hanging in the hall closet next to the front door, and me saying, "It's a bit chilly outside tonight for a walk. Let me get my night sweater."

## A BURDEN SHARED

My father died 31 years ago this month. In thinking about it, as I do every year, I remembered a sympathy card I got from a friend during that time. She'd written something about offering a ready ear and a shoulder to cry on if I wanted to talk. I wish now that I had saved the card because I cannot recall exactly the lines pre-printed in the card. It was something like:

> "A burden shared is a burden lightened; a joy shared is a joy enhanced."

When I sit down each Sunday to write this, I don't think about all the recipients until the very end. Before that, it's just me and the keyboard and the computer screen. The thoughts flow from my mind to my fingers, through the keyboard and up onto the screen, through my eyes back to my brain. Is that what I meant to say? Does that express what I'm feeling? Then I read what I've written again from the perspective of the readers. I often wonder how it will be received.

It is on Monday mornings, when I begin reading some responses, that I get my answer. It is then that my burden is lightened. It is as if, back in April, I was harnessed to a big cart full of rocks and told to haul it down the road ahead for an unspecified distance. As I work my way down the road each week it seems that on Mondays the cart feels a bit lighter because some of you file in behind the cart and help me by pushing. I can't see you behind the cart, but I can sense your presence. I thank you, individually and collectively, for the effort! Sharing this burden definitely lightens it.

Now for the second half of the quote from that card: "...a joy shared is a joy enhanced." I want to remind you that I'm also going to need your help enhancing my joy on January 11, 2003, at the Recreation Center in Sunnyvale, I'm going to have a "Light at the End of The Tunnel" party. If you've got something else scheduled, just come for a few minutes before or after. Stay for some food, join the circle(s) of dancers for a dance or two, share a hug. I say—if you've been helping push this load of rocks down the road, you should share in the celebration when the load of rocks gets delivered and dumped!

And I thank you all, collectively and individually, for your companionship during this journey. I would have done it without you, but having you accompany me has made a world of difference.

Loui

* * * * * * * * * * * *

# IN THE TROUGH OF THE WAVE

## Sunday, September 15, 3:30 PM

I have come to accept that this time in the chemotherapy cycle is the hardest. All the drugs have done their work and I'm left with the ravaged landscape, and repair work is slow to show. I am so dry! It seems that I am drinking gallons of water and I still taste like the wood from the south side of an old barn. But this too shall pass. Maude and Ralph will be sent in shortly and I'll be tasting the world's bounty come about Wednesday.

**CLIP-AND-SAVE TIME LINE**

If any of you know someone who is going to be requiring chemotherapy, here's a handy time line (assuming they have a similar two-weeks-on-two-weeks-off regime).

>Day 1-2 THE CREST OF THE WAVE:
>Chemotherapy begins. Assuming you get some anti-nausea drugs, you'll still feel fine.
>
>Day 3 BEDTIME FOR BONZO:
>Weak, sleepy, plan to stay in bed.

### Day 4-9 SLIDING DOWNHILL:
The situation deteriorates as the drugs do their work. The needle on the ol' Energy Meter starts dipping. The doctors call it mucusitis, but I call it Chemo-Mouth. Your saliva dries up, your taste buds die, your gums get tender, and your appetite falls away. If it gets really bad, you have mouth sores, difficulty swallowing, fungus on the tongue and, if you're really unlucky, the dreaded slime.

### Day 10 MORE BEDTIME:
Weak, sleepy, plan to stay in bed. The good news is you can't feel your mouth when you're asleep.

### Day 11-13 ON DOWN THE HILL:
Continued deterioration. Schedule more naps.

### Day 14-20 THE TROUGH OF THE WAVE:
Things don't get any worse, but they don't get better yet either. The drugs have stopped, but it takes 5-7 days for the white blood cells to show up and start repairing the damage. If you're lucky, you get Neupogen or Neulasta to jump start your bone marrow into producing the white blood cells. [This week is the hardest part of the cycle for me, waiting, being patient.]

### Day 21-28 UP TO THE CREST AGAIN:
You know the healing and recovery have begun because you'll feel that WHUMP-WHUMP-WHUMP sensation in your bones, which means the white blood cells are on their way. There will be daily improvement: bye-bye, Mouth Sores! Hello, Saliva! Welcome home, Taste Buds. Food, glorious food! And then you get to do it again….

*Loui Tucker*

## EYEBROWS

I miss my eyebrows! Now that I have no eyebrows, I have become quite the connoisseur. I caught myself in a meeting this past week staring at the eyebrows of the people seated around me: bushy eyebrows, thin eyebrows, arched eyebrows, flat eyebrows, salt-and-pepper eyebrows, uni-brows….

This week's giggle: I got hot and sweaty at a dance class and, while wiping my forehead, wiped off one of my eyebrows. Someone came up to me to say, "Umm, Loui, you've lost an eyebrow and you're looking a bit unbalanced. You need to either draw that one back on or wipe off the other one." (I wiped off the other one.)

## ME AND THE MIRROR

Rosh Hashana (Jewish New Year) was September 6 this year. Yom Kippur (Day of Atonement) is Monday, September 16. During the intervening days, Jews are encouraged to reflect on the past year, examine their deeds, mend broken relationships, resolve grudges and conflicts, ask forgiveness for wrongs committed, and forgive others who have wronged them. Quite a "to do" list!

On Rosh Hashana, my rabbi told the story of a wealthy miser. The wealthy man was directed to stand before a window. "What do you see?" he was asked. "I see people on the street," the wealthy miser answered.

Asked to move in front of a mirror, the wealthy man was again asked, "What do you see?"

"I see only myself," he replied.

"Aha!" came the explanation. "The only difference between a mirror and a piece of window glass is a thin coating of silver. The silver obscures our view of other people and we see only ourselves."

Cancer does something similar to the people it invades. I had read about how cancer makes its victims very self-centered, self-focused, and self-absorbed, but I always hoped it would not happen to me. We can't really help it, though, because we feel and see the results of the cancer and the treatment for it daily, even hourly.

I am reminded every time I shower and don't have to shampoo my hair. I am reminded every time I look in a mirror or see my reflection in a shop window. I am reminded every time I plan a meal because of what I can and cannot eat. Needing an afternoon nap if I'm planning on doing anything after 7:00 PM is another reminder. And then there are the daily pills, frequent visits to the doctor, blood tests, and so on.

Relief comes in the form of concentrating on work at my computer or some other mind-engrossing task, sleep, and dancing. Most of the time, what used to be a window looking out onto my world becomes a mirror, and I see only myself.

Because that window became a mirror, I have forgotten some important birthdays, anniversaries and other events. I have failed to answer e-mails and phone calls until I get a reminder—"Hey, I left you a message last week. Did you get it?" I have neglected to properly acknowledge gifts. In focusing on my own problems, I have forgotten that others have problems too—a friend dealing with a painful divorce, another with kid problems, several with work-related stress, one who was laid off work, yet another who has moved into a nursing home, and a valiant lady struggling with her own medical challenges.

So many people ask, "How are you doing?" or "How are you feeling?" Maybe that used to be a social nicety, but now people really do want to know how I am feeling. Either way, when I'm done telling them about myself, I have been forgetting that the appropriate next line is, "And how are you doing?"

Perhaps others will be quick to excuse me. "Loui, you're being treated for cancer. It's okay! Don't be so hard on yourself." Say what you like in my defense, but this sin of omission, the neglect of my friends who have been so supportive of me, is harder for me to accept in myself.

In the spirit of Yom Kippur I ask your forgiveness. If I have made you feel ignored or neglected, unappreciated or unacknowledged, I apologize. It may be a challenge in the remaining eight weeks, but I am going to try to scrape some of that "cancer-silver" off that mirror so that I can see all of my world and acknowledge and relate better to all the great people in it.

## EIGHT WEEKS AND COUNTING

Eight weeks? Did I just write that? Eight weeks!
Two weeks of rest.
Two weeks of chemotherapy (Round Five).
Two weeks of rest.
Two weeks of chemotherapy (Round Six).
That's eight weeks! Mid-November. I can see the finish line!

Then two weeks of rest and I start a month of radiation. What is involved in radiation? If what I am learning is accurate (and I have a LOT more to read), it means a short blast of radiation aimed at the spot where the cancer was removed, five days a week for four to six weeks. People who have only radiation for breast cancer (small localized tumor and no lymph nodes involved) report that it makes them very tired. They say it leaves you feeling wiped out, like you've just spent a day in the hot summer sun. On the other hand, those who have endured chemotherapy FIRST and then have radiation, report that radiation is a walk in the park by comparison. I'll let you know sometime in December.

I'm also reading that hair starts to reappear four to six weeks after chemotherapy stops, which means by the end of 2002 I should have a some stubble!

## QUOTES FROM FRIENDS

From Ken: "Cancer sucks. You're good. May the better team win."

## Dancing with Cancer

I have received lots of e-mail in response to my initial diagnosis announcement and the subsequent updates. I've gotten pages, I've gotten paragraphs, I've gotten sweet, brief good wishes. Ken's e-mail receives the prize as the most concise, precise, and to the point. I printed it and had it on an index card by my keyboard for a while. I still occasionally use it as a falling-asleep mantra.

> From Luane: "Hope is the ability to hear the music of the future: faith is the courage to dance to it today." (Peter Kuzmic, theologian and author)
>
> From Melissa: "In my mind, cancer treatment is a bit like flying—any landing you can walk away from is a good one."

Amen to that!

Loui

* * * * * * * * * * * *

# AT THE CREST OF THIS WAVE

## Sunday, September 22, 2002, 5:30 PM

This is the fourth week in the chemo cycle, the "good" week. I can eat just about anything I want, and I can taste it. My energy isn't back to normal yet, but I don't feel the need to nap every afternoon. This part of the wave is delicious and freeing, except for that little gray cloud hanging around the horizon because I start Round Five this Friday, the 27th. Until then, until next Sunday morning actually, I'll be feeling just about normal.

Last night I treated myself to some crazy comfort food: fried okra! Start with a dish of little disks of sliced okra, mixed with corn meal and egg. Fry it, stirring a bit now and then, and eat it hot with ketchup drizzled on it. My mother used to fix this dish when I was growing up, and I still love it…. Sabine doesn't like okra, so I get it all to myself. Umm, good!

I got another bit of good news about this coming round of treatment. Back in May when this all got started, I calculated ahead to the first weekend in October, when a wonderful dance workshop was scheduled. I determined it would be a non-chemo weekend, so I could attend the workshop and participate fully. Then remember back in the end of July, I had to delay treatment one week because my white blood cell was too low. That delay threw my schedule off a week and pushed this dance weekend into the second week of Round Five. Having a chemotherapy treatment just before the workshop would mean having one of my Stay-in-Bed Sundays, and the thought of having to miss an entire day of the workshop was depressing! I considered canceling, but kept hoping someone/something would intervene on my behalf.

I talked to my oncologist about my chemo schedule, told him about my desire to attend this dance workshop, and he agreed to let me delay the *second* treatment of Round Five until the Tuesday morning after I get back! I'll be able to attend the workshop as if I were on an extended first week. My appetite won't be great, and my energy level will be lowered although not at rock bottom, but I won't miss any time on the dance floor! Go ahead and ask me how big a smile this puts on my face!

## THOUGHTFUL PEOPLE

There is a local law firm where I have been working as a contractor for several years. I designed their estate planning documents program and I visit three or four times a month to do maintenance, upgrades, and fixes. This week they called to say there was a flu bug going around their office and several people had taken time off, returned, gotten sick again, etc. They felt it would be unwise, with my immune system so compromised these days, to expose me to their germs. I was so grateful for their advisory message. What a thoughtful bunch!

## "UNCLEAN! UNCLEAN!"

They used to shout "Unclean! Unclean!" at lepers as they were being chased out of town toward the nearest leper colony. I felt a little like those lepers this week when I was looking into private health insurance as an alternative to paying $400+ per month for COBRA benefits to maintain my medical insurance. I wasn't planning on switching coverage right away, at least not until I got a clean bill of health from my current doctors, but I thought it prudent to check into the pricing and availability. Because I am self-employed and have been for over 20 years, I need an individual health plan.

The bad new is that cancer survivors are not considered "clean" until TEN YEARS after treatment is complete! TEN YEARS! Until that ten-year mark is passed, virtually no insurance company will touch an individual with cancer in his/her medical history. At the five-year anniversary of your clean bill of health, some insurance companies will cover you at DOUBLE the standard rate. There are also some special and expensive plans that cover only accidents and catastrophic injury, but do not cover incidental or preventive doctor visits. Experiencing mild but frequent headaches? Worried about a persistent stomach pain? Want to see a doctor about a skin rash? Pay for it yourself. I was advised: (1) keep your COBRA benefits as long as you can afford them; (2) get a job where they have a group medical plan; (3) get married to someone with medical insurance.

Can I get medical coverage through Sabine? Not yet. The school district where she works does not, at this time, have domestic partner benefits, although it is on the negotiating table for the current contract. I can only hope all the chips will fall into place in the coming months.

## THERE IS PAIN AND THEN THERE IS PAIN

During my week in the "trough" I get impatient waiting for my white blood cells to fix my mouth and release me from the dry mouth and sores and tender gums. I go to sleep each night saying, "Tomorrow I will feel better." I wake up, check out the oral environment, and I sigh, "Oh, well, not today...."

When I get in that state, when I am impatient or feeling sorry for myself, I tell myself that, however annoyed I may be, this is still pain with an early expiration date on it. I know one day soon this will all be behind me. I remind myself that there are people who have pain that they know they will have for the rest of their lives. There are people dealing with arthritis and rheumatism and psoriasis and chronic back pain and bad knees. I think about the people living with HIV and AIDS. Theirs is a pain with an expiration date, but it's the same date as the expiration date on the sufferer. They deal with their pain every day, month after month, year after year. There is no light at the end of the tunnel for them.

These thoughts do not diminish my own pain. You cannot really compare your pain to anyone else's and it's not a competition anyway. However, these thoughts do make me raise my chin a bit, take a deep breath, put on the best smile I can manage, and get busy with my day. If they can get through each day then, damn it, so can I!

## BEST QUOTE THIS WEEK

From David:

> "Life is not measured by the number of breaths we take, but by the moments that take our breath away." (I did a google search and found one site that listed George Carlin as the author of this quote, along with many sites that provide the quote following by "author unknown.")

## WHAT TAKES YOUR BREATH AWAY?

Someday I will write an "Ode to Care Givers." In the meantime, I will tell you that there are times when Sabine takes my breath away. She puts in her full day as a teacher (which starts waaay before the students arrive!), plus all the after-hours meetings and paper grading and lesson preparation and phone calls—and she always has time at the end of that day for me and my woes. She offers me popsicles and milkshakes for my sore mouth. She suggests a walk in the evening. She fixes foods she knows I like and I can eat. Even though I've told her I can sleep through small skirmishes, she tiptoes around the house while I'm napping, worrying if the floor creaks or her printer

Loui Tucker

makes too much noise. She checks to be sure I take my pills. She starts a crossword puzzle knowing I'll join her and it will take my mind off my troubles. She kisses my bald head and tells me I'm adorable. She holds me when I need to whimper and complain and sob.

She is as constant and dependable as the water from a faucet. She is the vigilant night light that stays on 24/7. Her smile lights up my world and takes my breath away.

So, what takes your breath away?

Loui

* * * * * * * * * * * * *

# ON TO ROUND FIVE

*Sunday, September 29, 2002, 7:30 PM*

First of all, let me warn y'all that I won't be writing next Sunday. I'm going to be attending a wonderful dance workshop next weekend and will hopefully be dancing, dancing, dancing, instead of writing about my weekly doings. I'll be back in town Monday afternoon, but will be getting right back into my life with little time to write until the following Sunday, October 13. I'll be fine, so don't worry!

## ROUND FIVE, SITUATION TYPICAL

I started Round Five of the chemotherapy on Friday. The situation is the same as last month. Most of today, Sunday, was spent sleeping. I've got the usual dry mouth, poor appetite, no taste buds—you've read it all before. I don't expect much will change. Just don't ask me how tired I am getting of all this! The one positive note is that I just have to get through this round and Round Six and I'll be done! Six more weeks....

## WALK FOR AIDS

Sunday, October 20, 2002, I plan to participate in Santa Clara County's 10K Walk for AIDS, walking with a group of other small business owners. San Francisco has a huge event each year, gets lots of press and lots of walkers, but none of the funds raised come down here to our area. We have our own event, which raises money for local HIV/AIDS agencies such as AIDS Legal Services, ARIS, The Centre for Living with Dying, and the American Red Cross AIDS Project (there are actually nine agencies that will get funds). The funds are not for research. They are to help the people living with HIV and AIDS to cope with the medical problems, deal with the medical and legal systems, get emotional support for themselves and their caregivers, etc. I've written a lot about people suffering with terminal illnesses, daily pain, and far worse side effects than I have, and this is a way I can help them get through their days.

Sabine and I have walked four of the last five years (I was out of town one year) and want to do it again this year. I would like your support in the form of donations so I can help raise money for the charities that will benefit from the walk. Instead of schlepping a paper form around to all my dance classes and all the offices where I work, making my little speech, collecting the checks and cash. I am going to make it MUCH simpler for both of us. You can make a donation on-line, using your credit card. How easy can it get?

Here's the place to go: http://louitucker.chariteam.com.

That address should get you right to my web page, which is provided by and built into www.walkforaids.org (in case you want to visit and get more information about the walk). You can make a donation and see how the thermometer is rising as the donations are made. I hope to make my goal of $500, so every little bit helps. If lots of people make small donations of $10 on a credit card, it will add up quickly. Help me out, okay?

## QUESTIONS GET ANSWERS

Some of you write me questions, some specific to me, some general ones about cancer treatment. I figure of if *they* want to know, perhaps you all want to know too.

**Question**: Did you have a mastectomy and reconstruction? No, I had a lumpectomy and a lymphodectomy. The surgeon removed the tumor through a small incision on the armpit-side of my left breast, which left me with a small crescent-shaped scar and a small dent/divot/depression. I have another small scar at the base of my left armpit where he took the sample of my lymph nodes.

The only side effect I still have is numbness from my armpit to my elbow. There is a nerve that runs through that area and, in taking the lymph node sample, it is well-nigh impossible to avoid clipping the nerve. The surgeon told me it was like seeing a single blond hair in a piece of quiche and trying to take a scoop out of the quiche without cutting the hair. So the nerve usually gets cut and it take a while (months, actually) for the other nerves in the surrounding tissue to take over the function of the missing nerve. I have no loss of strength or agility or range of motion, just numbness, and it is diminishing as time passes.

**Question**: I heard you did some hypnotherapy. Did it work for you? Yes, I had four sessions with a hypnotherapist. The first three sessions were in May, before chemotherapy started. The first session dealt with the immediate pain from the surgeries. The next two sessions I asked for specific help going into the chemotherapy: I wanted to continue to feel strong. I wanted to maintain a positive attitude. I wanted a sense of serenity and acceptance. Rather than fighting and resisting and fearing the drugs, I wanted to welcome them, encourage them, see them as fighters working on my behalf. I wanted to avoid nausea, if possible. Then I had one more session after the chemotherapy started to specifically help me with the pain from the mouth sores and to help me sleep.

Did it work? There is really no way to test it. How would I have reacted if I hadn't had the hypnotherapy? Would I have felt as strong? Would I have had as much pain? Would I have had nausea? Would I have slept as well? I can't go back and do it again *without* the hypnotherapy. I certainly don't want to do this cancer treatment thing AGAIN and try it without hypnotherapy the second time around to see if there is any difference! I will just say that I don't regret spending the time and money on hypnotherapy because I believe it helped me.

**Question**: Are you still having the hot flashes or have they already gone away? The short answer is yes, I still have them, but the situation changes depending on where I am in the chemo cycle. When I am taking the Cytoxan, it blocks ALL estrogen production, so the night sweats are at their worst (I have almost no hot flashes during the day), very hot and usually every hour. They don't last long and I usually fall right back to sleep, but they are disruptive. Eight one-hour naps is not the same as eight hours of uninterrupted sleep. Then when I'm in the two-week recovery period, I get some relief because my body is allowed to produce what little estrogen it still can. The night sweats are less frequent, not as hot, and typically come at two hours (or more) intervals. Last week, right before I started Round Five, I actually slept four hours without an interruption.

I did try two different combinations of herbs (one Chinese, and one recommended by a local health food store). Neither seemed to make any difference and I had to take the herbs three times a day, which was a nuisance, so I stopped taking them.

## A RESPONSE THAT MADE ME CRY

Last week I asked, at the end of my e-mail, "So, what takes your breath away?" I got a lot of interesting responses, mostly having to do with loved ones—children, spouses, partners, parents, close loving friendships. This one was special:

> "Watching my 85-year-old mom, two-time breast cancer survivor, hold hands with her 80-year-old boyfriend."

Now there is something to aspire to!

Have a good week, everyone. Don't wait for e-mail from me next week. I won't be able to write again until Sunday, October 13.

Loui

* * * * * * * * * * * *

# DARN—ANOTHER SETBACK!

## Sunday, October 13, 2002, 9:30 PM

They moved the finish line again! Last Tuesday morning I went in for the second half of Round Five of the chemotherapy and once again my white blood cell count was too low. I even volunteered to get the treatment, take the risk of mega-sores in my mouth, even put up with the dreaded slime, but the doctor said no. He said the count was so low I'd be risking a hospital stay with a high fever. I had to wait a week, until this coming Tuesday, for the second half, which moves my finishing date at least a week. Sigh!

I can just imagine those of you wagging your index finger, saying, "See, you should not have gone to that dance workshop. You overdid it, danced too much, got too little sleep, ate all the wrong food, and that low white blood cell is the result!" And those of you who were at the dance workshop with me are probably remembering how much I danced, and are sighing in sympathy, regretting that I'm paying for my joy.

Well, the doctor told me specifically and repeatedly that no matter what I did at the dance workshop, it would not have raised or lowered my white blood cell count. In fact, to quote him, "In order to lower your white blood cell count, you'd have to be doing chemo drugs recreationally!" Yeah, like that's a possibility!? He also said this is fairly typical in the fifth and sixth months of chemotherapy. The bone marrow reserves are depleted and the counts just don't bounce back like the earlier months.

So, all this week I was in a holding pattern. I should have seen the omen: leaving San Jose for the dance workshop, we sat on the airplane on the tarmac for two very long hours waiting for permission from Chicago to take off (Chicago had major weather problems that morning and all flights were delayed). Similarly, this week I'm waiting to finish Round Five. It's like going for a long run and being just 200 yards from home. You can see your house ahead in the distance, and the hot shower with your name on it. You're hot and sweaty, your muscles are throbbing, your lungs are aching…but you're stuck at a red light, watching traffic race by, breathing exhaust fumes, waiting for permission to cross the street and run home.

I had been looking forward to writing this week: "I'm done with Round Five!" but I will have to wait until next week. Drat! This means moving the start of Round Six from October 25 until November 1 at the earliest, assuming my white blood cells recover from the Adriamycin this week. It also means that the second half of Round Six may also be delayed because the counts will not recover enough. My goal back in May was to be able to enjoy a Thanksgiving meal with fully recovered taste buds, but that scenario is looking less and less likely. I will be thankful the chemo is over, yes, but I don't know if the meal is going to be all I've been envisioning. Oh well….

**REPORT ON THE WALK-FOR-AIDS FUND-RAISING**

As I wrote two weeks ago, Sabine and I are participating in the Walk for AIDS this coming Sunday, October 20. The meter on my website shows $285 raised so far. I've also collected almost $100 in checks. Thanks again to everyone who donated! Every dollar helps. It's not too late to add your support. Drop by my website to donate on line: http://louitucker.chariteam.com, or you can always write me a check.

Sabine's birthday (her 40th!) is Saturday the 19th. We'll be out of town Friday through Saturday evening, and having dinner with her parents Saturday night. Then we'll be up bright and early for the

Walk on Sunday morning. Chemotherapy or no chemotherapy, I will *NOT* take the 5K shortcut; I'm doing the entire 10K!

## PEACH FUZZ

My recently completely bare scalp is now covered with something like a soft peach fuzz. It's light-colored, almost white, except in the back where it's a bit darker. I'm told it is only temporary, not the hair that will eventually grow back. It just shows the hair follicles are not dead, but are ready to rebound when the chemo is done.

## TREATS AND GIFTS

Sabine and I finally got around to seeing *My Big Fat Greek Wedding*. It had been recommended by everyone. If you have not seen it, go! It's great fun!

One of my crazier friends presented me with false eyelashes. Not discreet, lady-like eyelashes, either! We're talking outlandish, flamboyant, drag-queen-sized lashes. One pair is an inch long and black and the other is similar, except the tips are pink! I may never have the nerve to actually wear them, but opening the package and seeing them brought forth a whoop of laughter. Thanks, Irith! I smile every time I see them on the shelf.

Ann, a dancer in one of my classes, caught me mopping my bald head with damp paper towels. "This will not do!" she thought. She bought a nice hand towel, **embroidered my name on it** and presented it to me as a gift. No more paper towels for me; I'm much too classy for that!

## THERE IS FATIGUE, AND THERE IS WEARINESS

Cancer professionals talk a lot about fatigue, particularly in the last months of chemotherapy. I'm not sure fatigue is quite the right word. To me, fatigue means a physical tiredness. That's a factor, of course, but I don't feel any more fatigued now than I did the second month. What I feel is a weariness, a wish that this could be over. It is particularly strong this week, waiting to finish Round Five.

There was a cartoon in the newspapers this past week. A character in her last month of pregnancy, drawn huge with child, is sitting on the couch. She says, "I'm tired of being pregnant. I am ready to have this baby. Really, really, really, really, really, really, really, ready." Her husband asks, "Anything I can do to help?" Her answer: "Can you invent a time machine that will transport me two weeks into the future to my due date?"

That's about what I feel like. I am weary of this road. I'm tired of stumbling up hills, climbing over boulders, traversing the gullies, and always longing for shade and a cool drink. I long for the smooth pavement of my everyday existence back in March. I know I'll go on, I know I'll make it through to the end, but I confess that I am getting weary of this process. I am really, really, really, really, really, really, ready for it to be the first of December! Beam me ahead six weeks, Scotty!

## BEING AN INSPIRATION

I have often wondered why what I am doing is so inspirational to others. Inside of me, I'm the same Loui I always was, and I don't feel like I'm doing anything extraordinary. I'm just plodding down the path I've been given. Here was the best answer:

From Shoshana:

> "You're an inspiration because you are not just plodding along this road you've been given. Whether

it's a smooth, flat surface, or full of boulders, ruts, ravines, and mud, you're DANCING down the road!"

Fine, put on another piece of music. Let's dance!

Loui

* * * * * * * * * * * * *

# BAD NEWS BECOMES GOOD NEWS

Sunday, October 20, 2002, 8:15 PM

I went in last Tuesday to see how my white blood cell count was doing, assuming it would once again be high enough for me to get the second dose of chemotherapy. Nope, bad news: my white blood cell count was still too low. The count was a bit higher, but still not high enough to risk the drugs. My initial reaction was fear—that I'd be told to wait *another* week or, worse yet, I'd have to do Round Five over again and be delayed an entire month.

But the bad news turned into good news. The doctors simply declared Round Five over, gave me a Neulasta shot (like Neupogen, but only one time-released shot instead of daily shots) to boost my white blood cell count, and told me to come back in a week to determine when Round Six could begin. They couldn't wait another week to finish Round Five and evidently didn't think repeating another entire month will make a big enough difference in the overall scheme.

Assuming my counts rise sufficiently by this coming Tuesday, as is expected with the Neulasta helping, I can actually do Round Six *THIS FRIDAY* the 25th, back on schedule. (For those of you who are wondering why they didn't just give me the Neulasta shot last week in order to boost my white blood cells back then, they can't give Neulasta if they are planning on doing chemo within ten days, because it stays in your body that long and interferes with the chemo.)

If you've been keeping track, that means I could be done with the Round Six, the last of the intravenous drugs and last doses of oral chemo, as early as **November 7**. If I can't get the second dose on schedule because my white blood cell production fails me again, it might mean one week's delay, which would have me finishing November 14, but that is still two weeks from Thanksgiving, plenty of time to heal!

I am psyched! In a month I'll be in the last chemo healing stage, and getting ready for radiation. The finish line is in sight. Yippee!

## SABINE'S BIRTHDAY

For Sabine's birthday we took a leisurely drive down to the Monterey Bay area, had lunch, and walked to the beach and back. We checked into our hotel, napped and waited for our dinner companions to arrive. It was a wonderful dinner with good friends, followed by a fire in the hotel room's fireplace, and sweet dreams. The next morning we had breakfast with the same friends, and another walk on the beach. We did a little shopping, had a light lunch, and were back in the San Francisco Bay area in time for dinner with Sabine's parents (Mom cooked Sabine's favorite foods, of course) and the opening of her birthday presents. The 36 hours went quickly but were relaxing and rejuvenating. Which brings us to....

## THE WALK FOR AIDS

Sunday morning Sabine and I were up at 7:15 AM to get to the Walk for AIDS on time and register the money we collected. We both walked the entire 10K. The bottoms of my feet are sore, but that's about it. Not bad for someone in their fifth month of chemotherapy, huh? Combined, Sabine and I raised over $1200. Our thanks to everyone who contributed. Lots and lots of $10 and $15 donations added up quickly. You are a wonderful, generous group!

## EFFEXOR BEAT MY HOT FLASHES!

I heard from two different sources about women being given a combination of Benadryl and Valium for hot flashes and night sweats. Always on the lookout for something to get me through the night, I asked my doctors what they thought of this drug combination. They said it sounded like a rather drastic solution because it would put the woman in such a deep sleep she just wouldn't feel when the hot flashes hit. She'd still have the hot flashes, but she would be too drugged to wake up. And what else might she not wake up for?

They suggested that if the hot flashes were becoming a problem I might want to try a drug called Effexor. I looked it up on the web and found out all kinds of interesting things about it. (You can read about it yourself by doing a google search on "Effexor.")

Effexor was designed to treat depression and then it is typically used in high doses (75-375 milligrams per day). However, doctors found that in small doses (as little as 25-40 milligrams per day) it helps with hot flashes and night sweats. Hot flashes are believed to be triggered by the brain, and this medication attempts to improve the balance of chemicals in the brain, limiting the number and intensity of the flashes. Effexor belongs to a group of drugs called "serotonin re-uptake inhibitors." (Among the possible side effects? Dry mouth! Big deal—how much worse can that get?)

The studies said that almost 60% of the women said their symptoms were relieved by at least half, and that they saw results within a week. The last study done with 24 women receiving chemotherapy for breast cancer was done over a year ago. I wonder why nobody is talking about this drug? Why did it take so long for my doctors to mention it?

I did read some warnings about withdrawal from the drug when being treated in high doses for depression, but I don't know if there is a similar problem if you're taking small doses for hot flashes. I'm going to ask my doctors about that before I fall in love with this drug.

So I decided to give Effexor a try, and suddenly I am getting four hours of sleep at a stretch! When I do wake up it is because my body wants a change of position, not because of hot flashes. Instead of hot flashes, once or twice a night I have warm flashes. I feel too warm for the covers, not steaming or sweating, just a little too warm.

Cautionary note: I'm not taking any chemo right now, so the Effexor might not work as well when I have all the chemo drugs in my system too. Then there are the questions of how long I can or should or would want take this drug, who will prescribe it after the chemotherapy is done, will there be a problem getting off the drug, and how long my medical plan will pay for it (otherwise it's about $70 for a one-month supply). In the short term, I'm grateful for what I've gotten—better, more restful sleep the past three nights than I have had in months! I'll keep you posted....

## THOUGHT-PROVOKING CARD

Outside of the card: "Sometimes it helps to just close your eyes and imagine yourself in a happier place."
Inside of the card: "Sometimes it helps to max out your credit cards and actually GO to a happier place."

I am in a happier place this week, because the light at the end of the tunnel is getting bigger and bigger, the cheering of the crowd lining the way to the finish line is getting louder and louder, and I'm feeling the surge of the bottom-of-the-tank reserves rising to my aid.

Counting down: three more weeks!

Loui

* * * * * * * * * * * * *

# ROUND SIX—I'M ALMOST DONE!

## Sunday, October 27, 2002, 8:00 PM

Round Six started on schedule on this past Friday, the 25th. I'm almost done, folks, almost done! If my white blood cells cooperate, I'll get my last dose of Adriamycin this coming Friday, November 1st, and I'll swallow my last Cytoxan pill next Sunday! Just one more week of drugs! Just one more Sunday lost to sleeping. Just a little while longer living with this dry mouth and poor appetite and low energy.

I remember this conversation back in June:

> SABINE (hugging me, trying to boost my spirits): "Hey, you got through the first treatment. One down, just five to go."
>
> ME: "Five to go? Five more months of this??? I can't believe I'm going to feel like this for five more months! July, August, September, October, November... Waaaah!"

At that point, with the darkest part of the tunnel ahead of me, five months seemed soooo long! Now, with the light at the end of the tunnel looming large and bright, the five months seem to have whizzed by. The finish line is seven days ahead and I'm going to cross it with my peach-fuzzed head held high! You know the victory dance those football players do in the end zone? You ain't seen nothing yet!

This week my oncology doctors will give me a referral to a radiology clinic and I'll schedule the first appointment with those folks. My white blood cell count has to climb back up after this last round of chemo (helped by a shot of Neulasta and two weeks of recovery) in order to start radiation, so I hope to start that in late November or early December. I've been told to anticipate a month of radiation treatments—five days a week for four weeks.

## EFFEXOR ROCKS!

I wrote you last week about starting to take Effexor to diminish the night sweats to help me sleep through the night. This drug is usually prescribed for depression but has been found to work well in small doses against hot flashes and night sweats brought on by chemotherapy-induced menopause. I'm taking half the minimum dose that's given to patients with depression.

What a blessing! I can now sleep 6-8 hours at a stretch at night. My hot flashes have been reduced to warm flashes.

My doctors have reassured me that they can prescribe a year's supply of Effexor and my medical plan will continue to cover the cost after the chemo is done. They believe my ob-gyn can prescribe it after that if I still want it. Withdrawal should not be a problem because the dose is so low, but it was suggested that, after six months or so, I try taking the pills every other day and see how it goes before stopping altogether.

## ALTERNATIVE MEDICINE

I've had some people ask me why I didn't consider some of the non-Western medicine alternative therapies for cancer. There are multiple websites, reams of articles in health food magazines and health food stores, and scores of books that tout the benefits of various combinations of Chinese herbs, Native American natural medicines, Mexican tree bark and roots, recent medicinal compounds discovered by the Swedes—you name it. There are advertisements for cancer clinics all over the world purporting to cure you of whatever cancer you have with a specific cancer-fighting diet, meditation, visualization, and nature-based tonics. They abound with a basic disbelief in and mistrust of Western-style medicine, and offer non-surgical, non-chemical, holistic, all-natural alternatives.

So why not? Because I am my father's daughter. My father was a mathematician and statistician. He believed in numbers in whatever form—raw data, databases, tables, charts, or graphs. Me too. There is safety in numbers. I am reassured knowing that tens of thousands of women have had the same cancer and taken the same combination of drugs and radiation—and gone on to live long, cancer-free lives. The drugs I am taking have been designed to do what they do, it is known precisely how they work and what side effects can be expected, they are tested extensively, and the results are published. Hospitals and clinics that specialize in treating cancer publish their cure rates regularly. No hocus-pocus, no guesswork.

Alternative medicine seems to offer a lot of anecdotal evidence: "I was suffering from low energy and poor appetite. I took Compound XYZ and within weeks I was feeling great again!" Health food publications include articles by doctors who claim to have studied the effects of massive doses of Substance ABC and can point to dozens of satisfied patients. Dozens? I wrote to the authors of some of the websites about the herbal concoctions they recommended, and none could tell me *how* the substances worked, just that they had reportedly worked for others who had tried them. The alternative cancer clinics don't publish reports or provide data on cure rates.

Part of conquering a disease is believing in the medical choices you make, and I am happy with the choices I made. Sure, I wish there were cancer cures that didn't involve pain or side effects or months of baldness, but few diseases are cured painlessly. I am grateful that doctors today have the arsenal of cancer-fighting drugs at their disposal. I am in awe of the women who took these and earlier drugs, survived longer treatment with stronger doses, and suffered far-worse side effects. I am relieved to be living at a time when cancer is not the death sentence it was just a few decades ago.

And I, along with millions of others, dream of a day when cancer can be avoided altogether by some sort of yearly vaccine that can sweep through a body and kill just the cancer cells.

I hope to have more good news next week, and we can all do an e-mail victory dance. In the meantime, remember that life is a journey and friends are the gifts you pick up along the way.

Enjoy your journey!

Loui

* * * * * * * * * * * * *

# CROSSING THE CHEMO FINISH LINE

Sunday, November 3, 2002, 9:00 PM

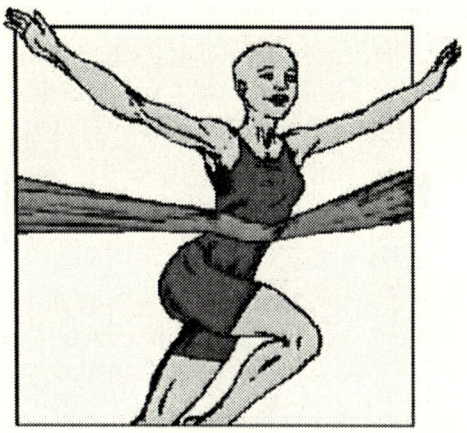

I did it! I had my last Adriamycin/5 Fluorouracil intravenous cocktail Friday morning, and I took my very last Cytoxan pill this morning. I am officially done with chemotherapy. I'm not feeling physically great right now, still tired from being asleep most of the day, but psychologically I am so high!

Tomorrow, Monday, I get two booster shots—one for my white blood cells and one for my red blood cells. Monday 10:45 AM Pacific Standard Time, I invite you to step away from your computer or lunch table or couch or whatever and join me in my Jubilation Jig: tappity-tappity-tappity-tap down the hallway, leap, spin, step-hop, turn. Then tappity-tappity-tappity-tap down a flight of stairs and across the lobby. Both hands wide to push open the double doors and leap, spin, step-hop, turn into the parking lot. Arms wide and yell: "WAHOOO!"

Then I have THREE WEEKS OFF! No drugs, no blood tests, no needles, no IV lines, no doctor visits for THREE WHOLE WEEKS! I have three weeks of R&R&R&R&R—rest, recover, renew, replenish, restore, revive, etc., etc. I will welcome back my saliva and taste buds and appetite for the last time, never to miss them again, and I'll start working my way through that list of foods I have missed these past months.

November 26, I have one more blood test to make sure my white and red blood cells are ready for radiation, which will probably start the following week. Radiation will be five days a week for four weeks, which pretty much takes care of December.

## PARTY COMING UP ON SATURDAY, JANUARY 11, 2003

If one more person says to me, "Gee, you ought to have a party to celebrate!" I'm gonna scream! Haven't you been paying attention? Do you need to increase your gingko biloba intake? **I AM HAVING A PARTY! SATURDAY, JANUARY 11, 2003, 6:00 PM 'til midnight.** Get out your PDA and put in the date. Mark your paper calendar. I'm talking about scads of great food and drink, balloons, lots of music for all kinds of dancing, songs, photographs, stories and anecdotes, hugs, poetry, a celebration to remember. Think of it as **Maude and Ralph's Retirement Party!** It's a big hall that will hold everyone on my e-mail list, plus all the folks to whom you've been forwarding the e-mail. (They are invited too!) Be there!

If you live outside the S.F. Bay Area, come for the weekend. A bunch of you can rent a van and drive up from S. Cal., enjoy the party, rent a hotel room (pretend it's dance camp!) and drive back down on Sunday. Or make it a long weekend: fly here Friday night, do some sightseeing on Saturday, come for the party, do a little more sightseeing on Sunday, and fly back home on Monday morning.

## IT'S A SMALL, SMALL WORLD

The scene is a bar mitzvah. The time comes to recite the prayer for the sick. A woman stands up and states my name for the healing list. A woman in the row in front of her turns around and says, "I know Loui Tucker the folk dance teacher. Does the Loui Tucker you know live in the Bay Area?" Not that remarkable, you're thinking. Well, one of the women in this story is from San Jose and the bar mitzvah was in Seattle near where the other woman lives. Both women are on my e-mail list.

This illustrates something my younger brother said decades ago (waaaay before the Internet shrank our world): "There are really only 400,000 people in the world and it's all done with mirrors."

## THE POWER OF YOUR SUPPORT

I look around my home and see evidence of your love and support: hats and scarves and wigs, books, jewelry, posters, paperweights, skin creams, wall hangings, t-shirts, plants, stuffed animals (my Chemo-Karate Bear now proudly wears a black belt!), memories of food provided and meals shared, photographs, and two file folders of letters and cards.

Your e-mails in response to mine have meant so much over these months. They have supported and strengthened me. They have made me laugh and cry. They have provoked further thought, inspired and motivated me. They have praised me and chided me and thanked me and teased me. I've gotten e-cards and photographs and jokes. You've shared your own stories, suggested websites and books, and offered assistance and advice.

You have all, collectively and individually, been a potent force in my healing. A mere "thank you" is insufficient. What has it felt like? Where will I find the words? It has felt like a warm, bright, sweet, tender, whirlpooling cosmic hug that surrounded and saturated me, day after day. Just as I wrote about the hypnotherapy I had, I cannot go back and repeat this journey through cancer again without these weekly e-mail/therapy sessions and see how different the experience would have been. I just have this belief that I could not have felt so strong, so cared for, so spiritually nourished without this connection.

I hope you'll stick with me for the next month or so, and get me through the radiation stage. I don't think radiation will be as traumatic or dramatic as the chemotherapy has been (I hope not!), but it will continue my learning experience. I'll have some pictures taken as my hair grows back and share them with you. I'll have pictures taken at the party and share them too. (What party? Haven't you been paying attention? The one on Saturday night, January 11, 2003!)

For now, I'm just jogging lazily around the track, the shreds of finish line tape trailing behind me. I'm tired, but thrilled that this part is over.

Loui

* * * * * * * * * * * *

# SLOWLY RECOVERING

## Sunday, November 10, 2002, 9:00 PM

Some of you may remember that the third week in the chemo cycle is the roughest. This final cycle was no exception. Psychologically I was elated to be done with the chemotherapy, but it has taken my body until today to figure out I could be physically happy too.

Last Monday night my mouth was extraordinarily dry and Tuesday morning the mouth sores started to reappear. I stupidly thought the Neulasta and NESP shots I'd just gotten that were pushing my body to create new white and red blood cells would protect me from the sores. I delayed getting treatment, but during the week the sores just got worse. By Thursday night I was finding smiling, talking, and eating were all becoming a challenge, and I was feeling pretty puny. I showed up at the doctor's office Friday morning expecting the blood test to show that valiant and long-suffering Maude and Ralph, my last two surviving white blood cells, had finally cashed in their chips and gone to the Great Blood Stream in the Sky. It was not quite that bad. The phlebotomist said I was merely, "…driving around on fumes." Anyway, a short while later, I left with prescriptions for a short round of antibiotics and a refill of The Stanford Mouthwash. Amazing stuff these drugs! I felt markedly better by Friday night and have been steadily improving. I expect to be out on the playing field very soon!

## HAIR IS APPARENT

The hair on my head is already growing back! I'd say the hair is…oh…about…1/8 of an inch long—but it's HAIR! I have incipient eyebrows and eyelashes too!

## FUN WITH FINGERNAILS

And you should see my fingernails! I have been treating myself to twice monthly professional manicures for the past couple of years. While I'm having my nails done, I usually just sit back and relax, sometimes with my eyes closed, and I have the habit of wearing a beige nail polish. I have not actually seen my naked fingernails for a long time.

This week my manicurist said, "Loui, have you noticed that your fingernails are striped?" It's like the growth rings on trees. As my nails have grown out during the course of the chemotherapy, the drugs have caused a slight change in the color of my nails, paler when the drugs were in my system. My fingernails appear to be striped (or perhaps banded is the correct word). I had my manicurist leave the polish off this week so I can show people. The effect is quite strange, and I don't remember reading anything about this little bonus in any of the cancer information literature.

I had Sabine take some pictures today. They did not turn out all that clear, but you will get the idea. Go to: www.louitucker.com/PostChemo.htm

## TREATS THIS WEEK

Pumpkin chiffon pie, thanks to Debbie and her mother. Easy on the mouth and yuuummmy!

## ALTERNATIVE THERAPY, PART TWO

After I wrote about my thoughts on alternative cancer treatment, some people wrote to ask me if I had talked to my oncologists about any alternative cancer treatments and what, if anything, they said. I can't quote them precisely, but here's the gist of it: Alternative treatment is misnamed. It should be called *supplemental* treatment. Most of it is either ineffective or benign. Only a small percentage is dangerous. If it will give you a psychological boost, or make you think you're doing something constructive and positive, go ahead and do it. It is not likely to hurt you, and psychology plays a big role in healing. The biggest danger comes if you stop taking the prescribed drugs or chemotherapy. Alternative therapies should be viewed as supplemental, not a substitute.

One doctor also recommended I visit www.quackwatch.org if I had questions or concerns about specific alternative cancer treatment. It is a fascinating website. There are more than just cancer treatments discussed, but the cancer treatment area is huge. I spent many hours a couple of months ago reading about the various purported cures and processes and the doctors that the site managers have investigated. Visit if you're interested.

I also remember the statistics from the computer program that my doctors showed me when I went in for my first oncology visit. The program is based on statistics gathered nationally over the past eight years from treatment centers dealing with all types and stages of breast cancer. According to their database, if I did nothing more than have the surgery to remove the cancer and the lymph nodes, did *no* chemotherapy, and *no* radiation, I had a 50/50 chance of surviving for five years. Obviously, 50/50 chances were not good enough for me, so I opted to increase my chances by taking the chemotherapy and radiation treatments.

Now, imagine a woman with breast cancer who is drug-phobic, radiation-phobic and generally dismissive of "Western-style" medical treatment. Alternative therapies would provide an attractive, plausible option, so she might decide on some combination of these alternative therapies. Assume that after five years she is cancer-free (remember she has 50/50 chance of surviving). She can then claim that the alternative therapies worked for her. Something to think about, huh?

## ANOTHER MISNOMER

While I'm thinking about misnomers, the other one that I've run across frequently in the past couple of months in books, magazines, web pages, and e-mail is the adjective "cancer-preventing." Whether it's a tea, a tonic, or a full-fledged diet, it should be relabeled, "cancer risk-reducing" because it is not "cancer preventing." Nobody knows what causes cancer, so it's going to be hard for anything to prevent it. Doctors and researchers and folks looking for cures know what amounts to risky, unhealthy behaviors when it comes to cancers, but not what affirmatively and verifiably prevents cancer. High-fat, low-fiber diets are certainly bad for you, but a low-fat, high-fiber diet alone will not prevent cancer. Eating any specific foods or combination of foods or vitamins or herbs will not protect you, though it may reduce your risk factors.

It's like driving habits. If you speed, weave in and out of traffic, drive after drinking alcohol, and generally drive recklessly, you increase your chances of getting in an accident. If you drive at a safe speed, maintain a safe distance from other vehicles, observe the rules of the road, and keep your eyes on the road and your hands on the steering wheel, you reduce your chances of getting in an accident. You cannot really prevent accidents. Accidents happen. Cancer happens.

## LEMONS FROM LEMONADE

I can tell you that, having survived the treatment, and looking back on the past six months, getting a cancer diagnosis was neither devastating nor life-shattering. It was certainly not pleasant and you know I got cranky and discouraged at times, but there have been other events I have had to handle that were far more unpleasant. I have managed to make lemonade from the lemons: I have learned a lot about cancer that I didn't know before, faced down a lot of fears, and found strengths I didn't know I had. I have felt the power of my communities, friends, and colleagues, and I have made new friends and re-found old friends. I have a new respect, even awe, of people struggling with far more life-compromising health problems. I have a new-found appreciation of my body, my blood, my hair, my saliva, and taste buds. I have confirmed the power of positive thinking!

Wishing you a healthy week full of good food and good times.

Loui

\* \* \* \* \* \* \* \* \* \* \* \* \*

# STILL HEALING

### Sunday, November 17, 2002, 7:00 PM

The Good News: The mouth sores are gone, and saliva and tastebuds are slowly returning. My energy and enthusiasm are climbing daily.

The Bad News: After all these months of chemotherapy and avoiding people with colds and the flu—I caught a cold! It's not a particularly bad cold, just a runny nose and a ticklish throat, but what a time to get it!

A lot of people have asked if losing my taste buds means I can't taste *anything* and the answer is—no, I can taste some things. Fruit and milk products are fine. I consume a lot of hot chocolate, tomato or noodle soup, avocados, mashed potatoes, puddings, and pasta. Almost everything else is blah and tasteless: bread, rice, most vegetables, meat (unless it is in tiny pieces and cooked to death and in a soup), desserts that involve a lot of flour and/or sugar.

It is kind of like trying to tune in a radio station that is just out of range. You hear a lot of static and the signal fades in and out. As my taste buds return, it is like getting closer and closer to that radio station. There is less static and the signal gets gradually stronger. Last night I made a yummy veggie stir-fry over rice and it tasted about 75% of normal.

## MORE ON STRIPED NAILS

My friend David saw the photo of my striped fingernails and did a google search. It appears that I have Transverse Leukonychia. It sounds horrible, doesn't it? It basically means "striped fingernails." Here's the link: http://www.sma.org/smj/97apr6.htm. I also heard from another cancer survivor who said she had the same striped fingernails but never connected it with the cancer treatment!

## FEAR OF THE UNKNOWN

In my e-mail last week, I said that my cancer diagnosis "was neither devastating nor life-shattering." One of you asked me about that. "You also mention that you had to face down a lot of fears. Was the possibility of death one of those fears?" I sent back a quick response, but it got me thinking more about the fears and anxieties I have had.

My dying of the cancer itself was not a big fear because it was made very clear to me from the outset, by my surgeon, the nurses, the oncology doctors, everyone professional with whom I came into contact, that I was not in any danger of dying. I confirmed this with various books and websites. Stage One breast cancer is curable about 97% of the time, with "cure" being defined as no recurrence of breast cancer for at least 5 years. The 3% is attributed to women with other medical complications (diabetes, lupus, stomach ulcers, etc.) or advanced age.

Initially, Sabine and I both had some fears about the surgeries. I had not had surgery since I had my tonsils removed when I was 8. There is that fear that something will go wrong and you won't wake up. After the first surgery went smoothly, that fear diminished, at least for me. I guess it was a matter of having confidence in my surgeon and his track record.

I was afraid of the nausea that I'd been told was an integral part of chemotherapy. That turned out to be a non-issue since I had almost no nausea and what I had was minor.

I had some fears about people's reaction to the word "cancer." There are still a lot of myths and phobias associated with cancer, and I didn't know if people would avoid being around me. I noticed many people were, and still are, unable to even say the word "cancer" in my presence, as if the word is spooky, or bad luck, or it might hurt me, but I haven't noticed anyone avoiding touching me or hugging me.

I had some fears about the hair loss, mostly about the reaction of people around me. Would I be stared at, and would I be comfortable with that? Would I hear unkind comments, and how would I react? Would protective parents grab their shrieking, pointing children and flee? Would my clients avoid hiring me because of how a bald woman in their office might look to *their* clients?

I was afraid I would be too weak to work and that would impact my ability to support myself. I was afraid I would lose business and therefore income because (in spite of all my efforts to keep people informed) my clients would feel I couldn't work due to the chemotherapy, or they shouldn't bother me because I had the cancer to deal with.

I was afraid I would be too weak to dance, which would remove a major source of joy, recreation, and stress-reduction.

I certainly developed a fear of mouth sores and mouth slime after the two months of chemo, but I eventually resigned myself to them. I knew they would go away, that it was just a matter of coping for a while, so I just braced myself each month and rode them out.

There are fears that we can avoid, like a fear of high places or a fear of flying. There are fears we cannot avoid. I remember a lesson from the group therapy I did in my 30s: feel the fear and do it anyway. That about sums it up: you have fears and worries and anxiety, but you do what you have to do.

## ONE MORE WEEK

One more week before I have to think about radiation. November 26th I'll have a blood test to see how my white blood cells are doing, so my oncologists can clear me for radiation take-off. New adventures await.

Loui

* * * * * * * * * * * * *

# APPROACHING NORMAL

## Sunday, November 24, 2002, 7:00 PM

This week was a week of rediscovered joys and delights:

I can lick an envelope with one swipe. A month ago, it took some concentration and four or five swipes.

I can feel my energy building daily. There is a bounce in my step, sparkle in my eyes, zip in my voice, zing in my attitude. A month ago, if I did two fast dances in a row, I'd have to rest. Now three fast dances in a row is no problem, and four is barely a strain. I haven't needed to nap in almost two weeks!

I went to the gym for the first time since July, did some upper-body strength training, and played some racquetball. Back in July, I decided that if I had an hour free, the time was better spent sleeping than lifting weights, so I have not been to the gym in all these past months. The sensation of muscles tensing and releasing was very welcome.

I sleep through the night almost every night. No more night sweats. Not so long ago, I was waking up every 90 minutes.

I can eat almost anything I want. Only meat and bread are still a challenge. I haven't had soup in over a week (after typically having soup once a day for months)! Some foods I can eat, but they don't taste quite right. I'll describe it as the gastronomic equivalent of looking at a scene through a piece of gauze. Looking through gauze, you can see shapes and colors, and you can tell that people are different from trees and clouds, but the images are all a bit fuzzy and dim. I can't always tell if it's the way food tastes or the texture or what. It just seems that some foods taste fuzzy and dim, about 80% of what I remember them to be.

Sabine says my breath no longer smells slightly metallic. She assured me, month after month, that it was not exactly a bad smell, just different. And now my breath smells normal again.

My mouth is almost normal to me too, only slightly dry, and I don't yet taste quite right to myself. My goal is to wake up in the morning and not be first and foremost aware of the state of my mouth. As I am waking up, my mouth is always standing first in line for attention from my brain: "I'm dry!" "I'm sore!" "I taste icky!" "My tongue feels swollen!" Whine, whine, whine!

You know those pop-up greeting cards? Or those books for children that have pop-up figures in them? You separate the pages and something that is folded between the two pages stands up.... Well, in my mind, my mouth stands out from my body like that. At some point, hopefully very soon, my mouth will just fade back into being another part of my body, with no particular claim to my attention. It will just be there, useful for talking and eating and whistling and kissing.

## CANCER HUMOR?

Needing a mental lift the other day, I thought I'd take a few minutes to search the web for cancer jokes. Yikes, was that a mistake! Lots of morbid humor and sick humor and stupid jokes and just plain not-funny humor. Many of them were specific to a certain type of cancer and also not funny. This is the one joke I enjoyed, even though it's a variation on the "Man on the Roof of His House During a Flood" joke.

> A woman with cancer returns to religion with fervor. She believes God will help her get better. Early in her sickness, a surgeon proposes radical surgery.
> "No," she says, "I don't want to get mutilated and suffer pain. It's not necessary, God will help me."

She also sees a radiologist but he proposes radiation to treat the tumor. "No," she says, "I don't want radiation burns inside and out. It's not necessary. God will help me."

A year later, the cancer has grown and metastasized. It's painful and she is referred to an oncologist. Chemotherapy is advised. "No," she says, "I don't want to be sick all the time and lose my hair as well. It's not necessary. God will help me."

She eventually dies. She goes to Heaven and demands an audience with God. "Why didn't you help me?" she whines.

"What do you mean? I sent you help three times: a surgeon, a radiologist, and an oncologist. What more did you want?"

## RADIATION IS NEXT

I go to the oncology clinic this Tuesday for a blood test. I hope to start radiation the first week of December. I know the first visit will be to get my tattoos. Yes, tattoos. Instead of trying to calibrate and position the radiation equipment every day (five days a week for four weeks), they set you up, get the correct position once and tattoo little head-of-a-pin-sized blue dots on your skin. Every time you come for a radiation treatment, they just line up the blue dots, zap you, and you're done. I've been told that disrobing and getting dressed again take longer than the actual radiation procedure.

I hope my doctors will also clear me for two other things. One is hot-tubbing, something I used to enjoy once a month or so. Perhaps I should be more specific: public hot-tubbing. If we owned our own personal, private hot tub, that would be fine, but the oncology clinic staff frowns severely on exposing a depressed immune system to public germs, no matter how careful and hygienic the hot-tub establishment claims to be. I presume, with my blood stream fully stocked once again, that Sabine and I will be allowed to use our gift certificates for an hour's soak at our favorite local tubs.

The other hope (now, don't laugh) is that I'll be cleared to clean the cats' litter box again (we have three indoor cats). Cat feces is supposed to contain some pretty nasty organisms and cleaning a cat box while on chemotherapy, no matter how careful you promise to be, is strictly forbidden. Poor Sabine has been stuck with this chore for the last six months and it's about time I got back to doing my job.

## MAKING PLANS FOR 1/11/2003

I'm making a budget and planning my January 11 "IT'S ALL OVER BUT THE SMILING" party. I'm thinking about food, decorations, music, entertainment, commemorative gifts, the works! I hope you're making plans to attend. By the way, kids are welcome, both the real kind as well as those "inner children."

Happy Thanksgiving (Thursday) and Happy Chanukah (starts Friday night). I have my appetite and taste buds all prepped, so bring on the pumpkin pie and latkes with sour cream!

Loui

* * * * * * * * * * * * *

# I AM A CANCER SURVIVOR, HEAR ME ROAR!

## Sunday, December 1, 2002, 8:30 PM

It was a delicious week! My mouth feels absolutely normal. I can sit for hours at a time without giving a moment's thought to the texture, moisture level, tenderness, or flavors in my mouth—a big change! I have my old appetite back, I have been able to eat, drink, *and* taste all the wonderful foods put before me, I have loads of energy, and I feel fabulous! This past week I ate lots of my favorite foods, and found a *new* favorite: pumpkin ice cream pie (pumpkin pie ice cream frozen into a pie shell). Thanks, Kathy—it was incredible! I also feel that I get so much more done each day because I'm not taking an hour or two out to nap in the afternoon.

When I went for the blood test last Tuesday I was cleared for radiation, hot tubbing, cleaning the litter box, and a prescription for Tamoxifen (more on that later). As a side light, my doctors said that, as energetic as I have been feeling, my blood chemistry says I am still running on about 2/3 of a tank. They seem to think I will be feeling even *better* over the next month or two. I replied that if I feel any better than I do now, I should invest in some lead-soled shoes because I'll probably start flying.

That last thought reminds me that I have also started dreaming again. I don't know whether it was the chemotherapy itself, or the disrupted sleep, or lack of deep sleep, or something else but, whereas I was once the type to have vivid, logical, memorable dreams fairly frequently, the past six months I didn't dream at all. Last night, I dreamt, as I used to, and in this specific dream, I could float and fly. I dreamt about rising, and I could see myself taking big steps that become sailing leaps until I was drifting above the treetops and rooftops. What a great feeling!

### HAIR'S TO YA!

The hair on my head is still very short. The dark, downy fuzz that started showing up the end of October has gradually fallen out, and what is growing on my head now appears to be thicker, coarser, and permanent. My hair used be sort of salt-and-pepper and I painted in the purple highlights. Now it appears to be mostly salt with a little pepper. Curly? Sorry, the hair is still too short for me to tell, although it appears to be growing in odd directions like I have a head full of cowlicks. Some of the reading I've done says that hair growing back after chemotherapy as a different texture (formerly straight hair grows in curly, formerly curly hair grows in straight) is rare. On the other hand, some cancer-support Internet sites say it is so common they have nicknamed it "Chemo Curl." I'll let you know in coming weeks.

### RADIATION

I am scheduled for my first visit to the radiologist on Monday, Dec. 9. I am on a waiting list for this week (Dec. 2-6) in the event there is a cancellation. That first appointment will probably be one of those "meet-and-greet" diagnostic visits where they review my medical file and x-rays and blood tests with me and tell me what to expect in the way of treatment. Then I'll probably have to schedule a second appointment for the tattooing session, and *then* I'll actually start radiation treatment on the third visit. I hope to actually be done with all the radiation before the big party on January 11, but I cannot be sure at this point.

In preparation for the radiation treatment, I've been doing my homework, of course. I found out more about *why* they do the tattoos. It is partly to line up the machines during the treatment. It is also so that, in the future, any radiologist can tell that you've had radiation in that area, because you can only get radiation once on any given spot. Also, if you get cancer in the other breast, the radiologist will be able to tell where the area that was radiated ended.

I also had been under the impression that the radiation is aimed straight-on at the breast and lymph nodes. Not so! If they did, they'd be radiating the lung on that side and, in the case of the left breast, your heart, which you want to avoid. The radiation is done on a tangent so that the radiation goes through the breast and out into the air.

When you are getting radiation treatment you have to avoid soaps that have fragrance, deodorants, or any kind of metal, all of which interact with radiation. You also can't use most standard-issue underarm deodorants, because they contain aluminum zirconium. Talcum powder is also out. I'll probably switch to cornstarch. I was also told there are some non-aluminum zirconium deodorants available at health food stores.

## TAMOXIFEN

After giving it some thought and doing some research, I've decided to take Tamoxifen, at least to see how I react to it. Why take it at all? It blocks estrogen (my tumor tested estrogen-positive). Also, Tamoxifen appears to change a cancer cell's normal growth factors. In other words, it tends to "lighten up on the accelerator and press on the brakes" (to quote Dr. Susan Love's book) at least in estrogen-positive tumors like mine. There are some preliminary studies that indicate Tamoxifen affects the immune system by increasing something researchers call "natural killer cells." Tamoxifen is recommended for women with my type and stage of breast cancer, and it is statistically effective in preventing cancer in the other breast (10-15% fewer incidents).

There are some potential side effects, of course, so I'll be on the lookout for problems. Stopping is always an option. Sabine's mother took it for the recommended five years, as have a few of my friends who had breast cancer treatment, and tens of thousands of other women. Side effects range from severe in a very few cases, to mild in fewer that 20% of women. The oncologists have said the hot flashes may get worse (because I'm taking Effexor, mine have been reduced to occasional warm flashes), and other typical menopausal problems may worsen. Tamoxifen also appears to create a slight increase in uterine cancers, and some women experience depression. I'll wait and see.

## NORMAL IS GREAT!

I remember a book in the '60s written by Richard Farina called "Been Down So Long It Looks Like Up to Me." My variation on that is "Been Up Long Enough It Feels Like Normal to Me." I have at least a week, and probably longer, to enjoy my recovery and all of my returning energy and joy. How sweet it is!

Loui

* * * * * * * * * * * * *

# THE LAST STEP: RADIATION

## Sunday, December 8, 2002, 10:30 PM

9:15 AM tomorrow, Monday, I see the radiation oncologist for my first appointment. That will be a review of my mammogram, surgery, blood tests and oncologists' reports, and I will get scheduled for the actual radiation treatment. I hope I can get started with that very soon, like this week. I'm tired of waiting. I want to be done. I feel like I'm actually already done, and this radiation process is just the last stamp on the paperwork.

### TAMOXIFEN

I seem to be doing fine on the Tamoxifen, with no side effects apparent after ten days. Okay, well, maybe my "warm flashes" are a bit warmer, but that's almost not worth mentioning. When I'm awakened at 4:00 AM feeling warmish, it's hard to tell whether I'm reacting to an internal estrogen-based heat or I just have too many covers over me in bed. So far, so good.

### MISCELLANEOUS MUSINGS

I don't really need shampoo yet, but Sabine bought me a bottle of my favorite orange-scented shampoo, just for the pleasure of the smell.

## Dancing with Cancer

I didn't realize how much my sense of smell was diminished through all those months of chemotherapy. I thought it was just my taste. I could smell a lot of wonderful food that I could not begin to eat, like popcorn, fresh bread, fried potatoes, and cinnamon rolls, so I assumed I was smelling everything. Now that I really *do* have all my senses back, I realize I was missing a lot of subtle smells, like chamomile tea and basil and tangerines and dish soap and furniture polish.

I also feel that, when I get to take a really deep breath, I am filling nooks and crannies in my lungs that have not had air in them for many months. My breathing feels deeper and the air feels richer and my lungs feel fully expanded again. I am pretty sure there isn't a physical difference in my lung capacity (wouldn't my doctors have mentioned it?), and this is just a psychological reaction to the freedom I'm feeling.

You'd think that gaining back the weight I lost would be easy and fast and fun. "Just eat lots and lots of your favorite fattening things, and you'll gain it back in no time!" I hear you say. It's not that simple. I have discovered that it is just as hard to gain weight as it is to lose it. If you want to lose weight, you have to reduce calories by eating less and/or expend more calories by exercising more. Safe weight loss is supposed to be two to three pounds per week. Safe weight *gain* should be about the same, so I have to eat significantly more calories and/or exercise less. Even with my normal appetite back and my taste buds in good working order, I'm still used to eating a certain amount at certain times of the day. I am also used to getting a certain amount of exercise. I don't know how to exercise less, unless you expect me to not dance at my own dance classes (not likely). I have to make a very conscious effort to eat more and more often and eat food with more calories. Just as you do when you are dieting to lose weight, you tend to fall back on old food habits and eating patterns. So far, I have not been very successful.

When I was in the middle of chemotherapy, the weight loss bothered me a lot. I felt I needed all my bulk and substance to withstand the power of the drugs and fight the cancer cells that could be growing in me. I worried that being thinner made me more vulnerable, and more susceptible to infections and complications. My thinner body made me feel weak, which seemed to be verified by the anemia and fatigue. Now that the chemotherapy is over and the fatigue and anemia are in the past, and I feel normal again, I don't even realize I'm thinner until I look in a mirror or check the number in the back of my pants. I know that I am physically much thinner, but I *feel* like I always felt. I feel like me again. Self-image is more powerful than reality! We really are who we think we are.

The hair on my head is growing in nicely. It's only about a half-inch long, but it's pretty thick. Sabine and my hairdresser both noticed that the very ends of the hair are curving instead of standing straight up, and they seem to think this means I'll have wavy hair for a while at least. With my eyebrows and eyelashes getting more noticeable, I look less alien. I'm still as hairless as a newborn everywhere else, however, and that is starting to worry me.

## THE PARTY ON JANUARY 11, 2003

The big "I'M DONE, I'M DONE, I'M DONE!" party is about a month away. In addition to this mention here, I'm going to be sending out in the next day or so a separate invitation and a request for RSVP. I need to start planning and budgeting for food and drinks, so I'm going to need a head count. It would be bad to plan for 150 and have only 75 people show up. Vice versa would be just as bad.

You can respond to this e-mail and just tell me you're coming and if you're bringing family and/or friends.

If you want your attendance to be a surprise, you can e-mail Sabine and tell *her* you're coming. She'll keep track of people who tell her and will give me the total number without revealing the names.

I'll be sending out, in a separate e-mail, all the specifics about the time and the location and directions, etc., but for now, just be aware that EVERYONE is invited.

Yes, you can bring spouses, partners, significant others, and children. If you are receiving this e-mail at work, particularly if you work in one of my client offices, and there are others in your office who know me, they are invited too. If you've been forwarding this e-mail to friends and family, they are invited.

This will be a Celebration of Life and Our Ability to Survive and we should ALL have good reasons to be celebrating!

Loui

* * * * * * * * * * * * *

# I WAS ABDUCTED BY ALIENS!

## Sunday, December 15, 2002, 10:00 PM

Getting set up for radiation treatment reminded me of those news stories in which some Kansas farm girl was reported missing for three days. In those stores, when she finally reappears, she tells a bizarre tale of being abducted by aliens and beamed up to the mother ship where she was subjected to examinations and poking and probing by bug-eyed scientists and had samples taken of body fluids and tissue, before being deposited back on earth. (More on that later.)

The office visit on Monday was pretty routine. I met with the radiation oncologist and a nurse who took my vital statistics, reviewed my medical history with me, and told me what to expect. There was very little I had not already read before. I was warned again that, about two weeks into the radiation treatment, I'll start to feel very tired. Been there, done that, and I know what to do: nap!

The bad news was I'm getting a total of 27 days of radiation, 7 more than I expected. I'll get 20 days of general radiation aimed from the vicinity of my right elbow and angled up across my left breast and into the left armpit. The 7 additional days will be from the vicinity of my left elbow with the radiation aimed up into the left side of my breast and the specific site of the tumor. In case you've already done the math, that means I also will not be completely done with by the time the party on January 11 rolls around. Too bad! I'll be close enough to finished, so I'm having the party anyway!

On Friday, I went back to the radiation department for the set-up procedure. They measure you and calibrate the machinery precisely so that the daily radiation process itself only takes a few minutes each visit. This set-up procedure was what brought up the memory of the alien abduction story.

First of all, it was done in a room about the temperature of a meat locker. The technician was wearing a turtleneck sweater and jeans and a lab coat; I was wearing only a thin cotton robe, which covered only those areas not exposed to the machinery. Brrrrr! By the time the procedure was done, I was a human popsicle!

I was on a thin metal table that rotated and tipped. I wasn't strapped down, but my head was in a cradle to prevent me from moving it and my left arm was in a two-part cradle that held it up and away from my chest. The lights were dimmed and the metal table was raised and tilted and adjusted beneath me.

The machinery was two big pieces that counter-balanced each other. Sometimes one was above me and the other was below me, and sometimes it was vice versa. There was a television monitor that showed various calculations as they were being taken by the equipment—24.6 cm, 18.2 cm, 4.5 cm, etc. Every few minutes the technician would leave the room and x-rays were taken. The machines would click, the table would twitch, and she'd return. She used tape measures and calipers, and wrote figures on charts. Then out came the magic markers and she started drawing on my chest and armpit and left side (it's a good thing I'm not ticklish!). She even took photos of her artwork with a digital camera!

The lights came back up and she got out the needle for the tattoos—five tiny dots, each about the size of a pinhead. That took about 10 seconds: position the needle, zap, re-position the needle, zap, and so forth. "Okay, you can get dressed now." Elapsed time: 45 minutes. No probing, no tissue samples taken, but it was as alien an experience as I have ever had!

## WATERY WORLD

It poured in San Jose on Saturday, and the power was knocked out for three hours in the afternoon. Rather than attempt reading by candlelight or gray window light, Sabine and I decided to brave the weather and take a walk. We bundled up in hooded raincoats over our sweatshirts, sweat pants, and tennis shoes and headed out the door. We stayed dry enough at the beginning but then we got to a corner where the storm drain had become clogged with leaves and the street was flooding. Being civic minded, we rolled up our sleeves and pulled piles of wet leaves out of the drain until the water flowed again. It was very satisfying seeing the water level in the street drop as the gutters cleared and the water flow smoothly again.

So we walked down the street and repeated the procedure at the next corner, and the next, and the next. Eventually we stopped trying to keep our coats and pants and shoes dry and just sloshed blithely around in the water. It wasn't all that cold and the wind wasn't blowing (yet). We were pink-cheeked and laughing, and sweating inside our raincoats. It was so much fun! Then the wind picked up speed and started seriously pushing the rain around, so we decided to head back. By the time we got home, only our sweatshirts and the very tops of our sweat pants were still dry. The bottoms of our sweat pants were so heavy with water the pants were trying to drag themselves down off our hips. It felt so good to peel off all that wet clothing and hop into a hot shower!

Later, as I sat sipping hot chocolate, I reflected that, as little as six weeks ago, I would not have dreamed of spending the afternoon walking in the rain and cleaning wet leaves out of storm drains with my bare hands. How quickly my life has returned to normal!

Loui

* * * * * * * * * * * * *

# RADIATION BEGINS

## Sunday, December 22, 2002, 8:00 PM

Examination by the aliens continued this week, which is to say that radiation began in earnest. The drill goes something like this:

In a dressing room, I strip to the waist and put on a short cotton hospital gown. I walk down the hall to the radiation room. The room is, as you may recall from last week's description, the temperature of a meat locker. Fortunately, radiation treatment takes about eight minutes, so I'm not cold for very long. I pull off the left side of the gown to expose my left arm and chest area, and lie down on the cold metal table, my head on its cradle and my left arm in its cradle.

I have to remain absolutely motionless while three technicians scurry around me, calling out measurements, manipulating the table (which raises, lowers, tilts, and rotates), positioning the radiation equipment, and lining up the red laser lines with the tattoos. They use a magic marker to enlarge the tattoos and draw lines between them because the tattoos are tiny and don't show up well in the darkened room. Upon agreement that everything is set correctly, they slip out of the room and there is a 10-15 second long buzzing. I don't feel anything except cold.

The positioning, leaving the room, and the buzzing are repeated three more times. Why three more times? The first blast is done from above my right elbow up across my left breast and into my left armpit. The second is the same trajectory but from the opposite direction, from a position under my left shoulder. The third is aimed at the lymph nodes near my left shoulder blade and the fourth is aimed at the lymph nodes to the left side of my collarbone.

They have to be careful not to over-radiate or radiate something that's not supposed to get radiation at all. To do this, there is a slot in front of the radiation gun. Into that slot goes a thick clear plexiglass sheet about a foot square with a small, odd-shaped chunk of silvery metal attached to it. The technicians position the chunk so that it shields, for example, the thyroid gland when they radiate the lymph nodes next to my collarbone.

One of the side effects of radiation is a skin reaction similar to sunburn. (Radiation doesn't involve ultraviolet rays, so it isn't sunburn, and using a sunscreen lotion won't work as a preventative.) From what I've read, the possibility of burning does not correlate at all to one's tendency to tan, freckle, or burn from sunlight. Some patients burn and some don't. Everybody recommends applying liberal amounts of aloe vera to soothe the skin during radiation treatment, but if you burn, you burn.

I may have gotten lucky in one small aspect in that my radiation treatment coincides with Christmas and New Year's Day. Under normal circumstances, I'd get radiation five days a week for 5½ weeks. Because the hospital staff gets Christmas Eve, Christmas Day, and New Year's Day off, my schedule will be three days the first week (the one I just did), a three-day Monday-Thursday-Friday week (Christmas week), and then a four-day Monday-Tuesday-Thursday-Friday week (New Year's week). That means I'll get the first 10 radiation doses over a three-week period instead of over two weeks, giving my skin time to rest more between the blasts of radiation, which may decrease the likelihood of burning. The remainder of radiation treatment will be the more typical, five-day weeks.

So far (three treatments), I haven't had any reaction at all—no reddening, no tenderness, no rash, nothing.

## BBC and ABC

I remember hearing some women explain that they mark time by the birth dates of their children. For them, a memory might be described as being "before Charlie was born" or "after Pat was born, but before I got pregnant with Chris."

I think for women who survive breast cancer there is something similar. The year a woman fights breast cancer becomes a line of demarcation, and all events are remembered relative to that line—Before Breast Cancer (BBC) and After Breast Cancer (ABC).

## AN OPPORTUNITY FOR PERSONAL GROWTH

Some years ago, I was in a group that was preparing to take a five-day trip down the Colorado River. Part of the preparation was being informed how the Porta-Potty system worked. There were some grimaces and raised eyebrows and smirks as we envisioned a week of sharing a small and primitive chemical toilet with 15 other people. During a brief lull, one of the group members spoke up with what would become an important phrase in my life: "Okay, gang, just think of this as an opportunity for personal growth."

I have used this phrase many times over the years when faced with some task or event I thought would be tedious or distasteful or worthless. It didn't take long before using the phrase made me smile because I was reminded of the times I actually learned something valuable from an experience I assumed would be best forgotten.

This also brings up for me the words of the various breast cancer survivors who talked to me right after my diagnosis last April, before the chemotherapy started. They said something like, "Oh, I'm so sorry to hear you're going to have to go through this. I can tell you from my experience that it isn't pleasant. You'll be tired, your body won't feel right, you'll lose your hair, you may have to deal with nausea, you'll feel like the six months will never end—but you'll get through it and you'll be fine."

I hope, when I have the opportunity in the future to talk to women who've been diagnosed with breast cancer, that I can say something similar to them. And then I will add, with a smile: "Think of this as an opportunity for personal growth." Every cancer is different, some more life-threatening than others, but we each have the ability to take a firm and positive stand on our own behalf.

Loui

* * * * * * * * * * * * *

# THE HOME-FIELD ADVANTAGE

Sunday, December 29, 2002, 9:00 PM

Radiation continues, 8 treatments out of 27 so far. No skin reaction at all, but I was told that the majority of patients don't show signs of radiation burn until the end of the third week (12-15 treatments). I changed from a noon radiation appointment, which really disrupted my day, to an 8:15 AM appointment, which is not easy because I am not a morning person, but I'll do it for the next four weeks just to get it over with and get on with my day.

Someone wrote and asked if the radiation treatment center is only for breast cancer patients. No, this one is for all kinds of radiation, just as the oncology clinic I went to was for all kinds of cancers. Both facilities appear to treat only adults, but there are just as many men as women.

I went to the oncology clinic for my two-months-post-chemo checkup. My blood test showed my blood counts (red and white cells) are almost back to normal, roughly 97% of what they were when I started cancer treatment seven months ago. My white blood cell count is expected to drop in the next month due to the radiation, but not as much as during the chemo. The doctors were pleased enough with my overall recovery to set my next appointment out three months from now.

And I'm feeling great, I can tell you that! I have scads of energy, my appetite is back in full force and effect, and food is glorious (though I've only managed to gain back three pounds). I can wear mascara and I wash my hair every day now!

## MY FIRST HAIRCUT IN MORE THAN SIX MONTHS

When people see me only once a week or so, it seems to them that my hair is growing back very quickly, but from my perspective, looking in the mirror every day, my hair is coming back at glacial speed. It's quite silvery on top, but much darker in the back. Then Sabine mentioned Saturday that the neckline was looking a bit ragged, so we walked over to The Back Lot (where I had the Head-Shaving Party back in June) and I got a "clean-up" from Brian. I'll see if I can take, and post, some photos this week.

## VERY DELAYED SIDE EFFECTS

I was warned by the radiologist about a possible late-appearing side effect that can scare an unaware cancer patient. I read up about it and verified it does happen fairly often. The pectoral muscle under the breast gets radiated to some extent and when that muscle regenerates and heals, it feels quite sore, like you've done waaaay too many chest presses. The problem with it is that it typically doesn't show up until 3-6 months after radiation is over and you aren't thinking about side effects any more. Lots of women feel the pain and fear the cancer is already back and they panic! If I start complaining about chest pains in May, remind me of this, okay?

## THE HOME-FIELD ADVANTAGE

When an athletic team goes out of town for a game, the individual players have to cheer and applaud each other's efforts, and they have to generate their own motivation and will to win. The crowd at the stadium sees them as the enemy and certainly does not greet their talents and achievements with any enthusiasm.

But when that same athletic team comes home for a game, the fans in the stands are awesome. Teams love to play for the home crowd, because they feel bolstered and supported by all the noise and signs and excitement. Teams tend to win more games at home than on the road because of this, and it is referred to as the "home-field advantage."

I feel like I've had the home-field advantage against cancer for the past seven months. My fans in the stands and all the ones lining the streets at the finish line made my heart light and spirits sore. The e-mails and cards and gifts strengthened and encouraged me the same way clapping and foot stomping and cheers spur a team to victory.

I feel so lucky to have had the homefield advantage. So, family, friends, and fans, thank you!

## GEARING UP FOR THE BIG FINISH

Okay, so the party is on for the 11th and the head count is impressive—150-ish!

> Hall? Check.
> Food and drinks? Check.
> Decorations? Check.
> Singer? Check.
> Music? Check.
> Still gotta work on the t-shirts....

This is going to be so much fun!

By the way, I'll probably discontinue this weekly personal-therapy-session-mass-e-mail the end of January. I will write a report for all the folks who can't make it to the big celebration on the 11th, and I'll post some photos of the festivities. After that, I will drop y'all a line if anything startling occurs in the cancer department, but I hope my life becomes so deliciously boring by February that I can just kick back and read a good book on Sunday nights.

Loui Tucker

When the dust settles, perhaps I'll honor the suggestion made by many of you and try to get all the e-mails I wrote pulled into some sort of book for publication. Anybody know a literary agent?

Happy New Year to you and yours. Life is sweet, so take big bites and savor it!

Loui

* * * * * * * * * * * * *

# PARTY TIME!

## Sunday, January 5, 2003, 9:00 PM

The first side effect of radiation finally showed up. I developed a red blotchy rash on my chest, like a swarm of ant bites. At first, it did not itch. When I showed the rash to the radiation team and commented that the rash did not itch, they said, in unison, "Yet!" My doctor, of course, said exactly the same thing. Sure enough, two days later, the rash started itching. It's just a mildly distracting itch, not one of those itches that makes your eyes bug out in frustration. Applications of cortisone cream are enough to keep my fingernails away.

I've been warned that the next typical side effect, radiation fatigue, is coming soon. Bring it on! I can handle it!

The doctor said I'm probably looking at a total of 30 days of radiation, not the original 27 he had planned. This past Friday, I finished Treatment #11. Nineteen more to go. If my calendaring is accurate, I'll have my last radiation treatment on Jan. 30.

### SCARY MEDICAL DETAIL

Radiation is measure in "rads." Your average x-ray is a fraction of a rad. Radiation for purposes of killing cancer cells is over 4,500 rads. Yikes!

Loui Tucker

## PHOTO UPDATE

For those of you who don't see me regularly, I've posted a photo on my website that shows the current status of my hair. Go to: www.louitucker.com/PhotoJan0303.htm

## THE END OF THE CAMPAIGN TRAIL

When a candidate for public office finishes a campaign, whether it's a win or a loss, the candidate throws a big bash for all the campaign workers, staff, volunteers, and supporters. It's the most efficient and effective way of saying thank you. Having considered that image, I see the party coming up this Saturday as my way of thanking my "campaign workers." Okay, the analogy isn't perfect. Candidates shake hands, kiss babies, and make speeches. I took toxic drugs, slept a lot, and wrote e-mails. What I mean is that I won my campaign against breast cancer and it was not without the tireless efforts of my care givers and supporters. Just as candidates have people working behind the scenes for them, stuffing envelopes, answering phones, and walking door to door distributing campaign literature, I had hundreds of people thinking positive thoughts, saying prayers, writing cards and letters and e-mails, sending little gifts, and caring about every side effect and symptom. It's time to bring the campaign to a close, celebrate victory, and thank all the workers!

Some of you have questioned the wisdom of spending scoodles of money on a party at a time like this. Well, if I'd been paying for the medical treatment out of pocket, I wouldn't be able to afford it, but medical insurance took care of my treatment. If I'd been so disabled by the chemotherapy that I could not work, I wouldn't be able to afford the party either, but I was able to continue at about 80% of my usual workload, so that's not an issue either. Sure, it's expensive to throw a party for 150+ people, but I can't think of anyone who deserves a celebration more than we do!

*Dancing with Cancer*

By the way, in addition to the food and all kinds of dance music, the party will include a woman who does balloon twisting into the most amazing shapes, and a face painter and henna artist. And save room for the end of the buffet table: chocolate fondue! Wait 'til you taste homemade Rice Krispy squares dipped in hot dark chocolate!

### WE ALL NEED GOALS

I heard a song on the radio recently that had a line in the chorus that went: "I ain't never had too much fun!" This Saturday night I hope you'll join me and see if it is possible to have too much fun.

For those of you who cannot make it (I wish you could be here!), I'll have a report, probably with some photos, next week.

Loui

* * * * * * * * * * * *

# SO, HOW WAS THE PARTY?

### Sunday, January 12, 2003, 9:00 PM

Wow, was it ever a party! Someone did a head count at 9:00 PM when I was talking, and he reported there were over 380 (which is waaaay over what the sign on the entry way says is permitted by the Fire Marshall)! We danced and we ate and we hugged and we had a terrifically good time. The energy and excitement in the room pushed the needle right off the edge of the meter. I looked up a couple of times to check if we were creating stress fractures in the ceiling beams. I met some of the people I knew only through my e-mail exchanges with them. Several people had cameras, and I hope to get copies of some of the photos so I can post them for you to see next week.

The dancing was awesome! I teach both international and Israeli dancing, so dancers from all three classes mingled and mixed during the evening. When a Romanian or Turkish dance was played, the international dancers formed the inner circle and the Israeli dancers copied the dance movements in an outer circle. When the music switched to an Israeli dance that the international dancers didn't know, the dancers and their roles in the inner and outer circles reversed. If an Israeli song came on that both groups knew, the dance floor turned into a human Cuisinart with everyone jumbled together. Then there would be a slow dance or a waltz or a swing number and those at the party who don't come to my dance classes got up to add their bodies to the mix.

And then there was the food! Sharon and Zan Kleinman of Shazan Catering orchestrated the buffet table, and I use the word "orchestrated" because it was a symphony of food. They prepared and brought the bulk of the fantastic food, and made the buffet table look elegant and bountiful, plus they left room for whatever food was brought by guests, such as the 300 (I am not kidding and that is not a typo—300!) oatmeal raisin cookies. Donna Frankel took me seriously when I wrote back in July that I was dreaming of oatmeal raisin cookies, and she spent a week baking enough for the party. Fortunately, I got the last dozen or so to take home to enjoy. The chocolate fondue, as I anticipated, was a big hit.

Madelon Battaeiger and Nancy Dalton of Twistin' Shout Balloons fashioned balloons into three rainbow arches over the buffet tables plus six huge rainbow-colored balloon bouquets around the room. At the entrance to the hall, they created two balloons sculptures labeled "Maude" and "Ralph," my two very famous, very valiant, and long-suffering white blood cells. During the first two hours, Nancy made balloon sculptures for anyone who asked, and Madelon did some extraordinary face painting and henna art. Everything was so colorful and beautiful!

The t-shirts! I knew I wanted to make t-shirts to give away to commemorate the party, and I had been racking my brain for either words or art to put on the front. The design finally came to me around the middle of December and, after incorporating a change suggested by Sabine, I presented the concept to Susan Gregory who drew it for me. It is amazing the way she can turn a verbal description of a concept into a picture! Keep in mind that Susan works full time, dances at least four days a week, and makes doll clothes in her spare time, and she still found time to do the artwork for the t-shirts for me. The finished artwork went to Cathy Gill of By The Bay Advertising Specialities who found me a great deal on navy t-shirts and got them printed in less than a week! I've posted a print of the design at www.louitucker.com/TshirtJan03.htm if you'd like to see it. I only had 100 shirts made, and they were snapped up like everyone had been walking around naked. I had the folks who didn't get a shirt and wanted one write their names on a list, and I'm going to have another batch of shirts made for them.

Peter Bunny is the professional singer I hired to sing some songs for me. Peter goes one step beyond the average hired vocalist who just sings from his or her prepared list of songs. I asked Peter to learn two songs for me and he was more than happy to do so. The first was "I Hope You Dance," which was my gift to the assembled masses.

I gave a little speech before the songs, thanking the people who are written about in the paragraphs above and explaining why I chose the songs. Someone who came to the party too late to hear what I'd said asked me to write down what I said in this report. Since I was speaking unprepared and off-the-cuff, I can't reproduce what I said word for word, but I'll give you the gist of it, or at least what I would have liked to have said had I actually taken the time to prepare something.

"While I have never been a particularly private sort of person, I never imagined when I got cancer that I would be writing a weekly e-mail to 250+ people who would learn the intimate details of my mouth sores, appetite, weight loss, and pill regimen. And yet, it was the smartest accidental decision I've ever made, because it ultimately proved to be instrumental in maintaining my sense of well-being and my positive outlook. Because of that weekly e-mail connection, during the past nine months, I had the daily joy of opening my e-mail program and finding an inbox full of love and support. Instead of spam, chain letters, and old jokes, I got e-mails expressing concern and good wishes, and asking thoughtful questions and sharing positive comments. It was so uplifting and empowering! It was like a daily emotional vitamin pill.

"There are people who get a cancer diagnosis and tell very few people outside their immediate family. They don't want anyone at work or their church or synagogue or even the folks at the grocery store to know. When they hide their lives like that, they are missing out on the astonishing power of human connection. Despite what the media might be saying, that we are becoming more isolated and alone and disconnected, I know now from this experience that we really are all powerfully connected. Given the slightest chance, people will connect and share and bond, and I can bear witness to the strength of that connection. You became, individually and collectively, a sensational support group, and I thank you.

"So, this song is for you all, with my thanks and love. It is called 'I Hope You Dance' and was sung by Lee Ann Womack. Although the chorus says "I hope you dance," the song is more about taking risks and having hope and being positive and seeing the glass as half full instead of half empty and cracked." (I'm going to add the words to the song at the end of this e-mail.)

"The other song I asked Peter to sing is for Sabine, my partner and care giver.

"First, though, I want to announce to those of you who did not hear about it already through the grapevine: On January 2, 2003 (and for anyone interested in numerology, that's 01-02-03!), Sabine and I signed and filed the paperwork with the State of California so that we are now officially recognized as domestic partners. This registry is largely symbolic, because there are only a few rights and responsibilities involved, but it was a symbol that was important to us, and it's the closest Sabine and I can legally get to marriage at this point.

"So, Sabine was my care giver and I have tried repeatedly over the past months to thank her and tell her how grateful I am that she has been so supportive and good to me. She just shrugs her shoulders and shakes her head and says something like, 'Oh, don't be silly.

Anyone in my position would do the same thing. That's what we do for the people we love, we take care of them in times of crisis.' But you all know there are those who abandon a spouse, a partner, a loved one, either emotionally or physically, when they get sick, whether it's cancer or Alzheimer's. The fact remains that Sabine did have a choice, and I am thankful that she chose to stay with me and take such good care of me.

"There were two days spent waiting in hospital waiting rooms while I was unconscious in surgery, innumerable doctors visits, and watching while oncology nurses stuck me with needles and pumped me full of toxic drugs. She kept track of my medications, tempted me with food to keep my weight up, and tiptoed around the house when I was napping. She put up with my whining and complaining and obsessing. She hugged me and encouraged me, and kept me positive and focused on the future when I would be well again.

"This song I have asked Peter to sing was made popular by Anne Murray and it's a waltz. Sabine and I are going to dance to it and we want you all to get up and waltz with us. This song has been a favorite of our for many years.

"This is for Sabine, to say thank you for being my partner, for being my care giver, for loving me, and for allowing me to love her. The song is, 'Could I Have This Dance for the Rest of My Life.'"


And then we danced.


There was also a (unplanned by me) presentation by Etti Tassa and Kathy Knopoff. Etti had organized the collection of money from an astonishing number of dancers who shared the cost of a gift certificate for an embarrassingly large sum to a decadent hotel and spa north of San Francisco. Sabine and I were in shock when we opened the envelope. We hope to make use of it this spring. I didn't expect any gifts, but one of the tables was soon collecting cards and small packages and bouquets of flowers. It began to look like the gift table at a wedding reception. What a generous bunch of people inhabit my world!

It was an evening and an event I will remember for many, many years. It was like a glorious home-coming after a nine-month journey down a wretched patch of road. The party was everything I planned and hoped for and daydreamed about since its conception in July. I wanted a celebration of life, and I sure got it! Thank you all so much for everything!

Loui

\* \* \* \* \* \* \* \* \* \* \* \* \*

*The T-Shirt Design*

# Pictures from the Party

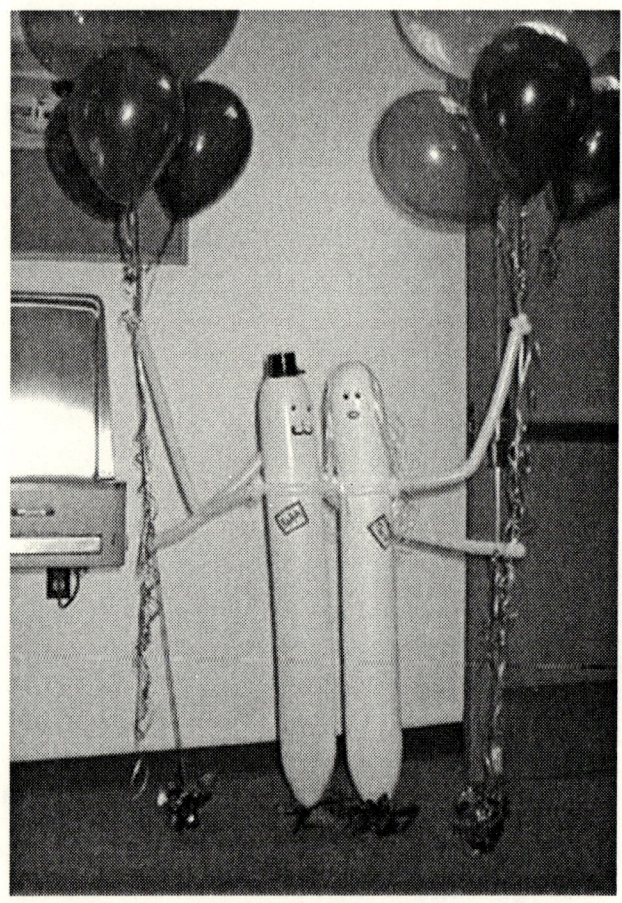

*Ralph and Maude*

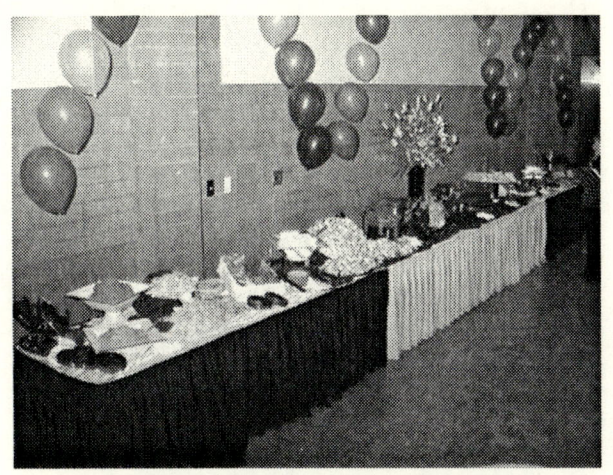

*The Buffet Table*

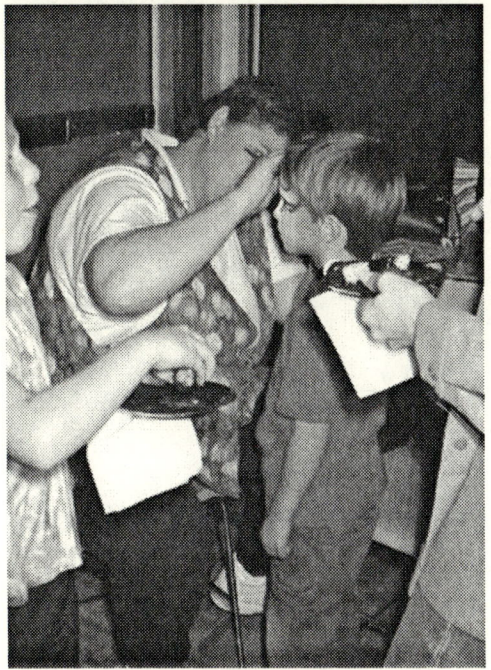

*Face Painting*

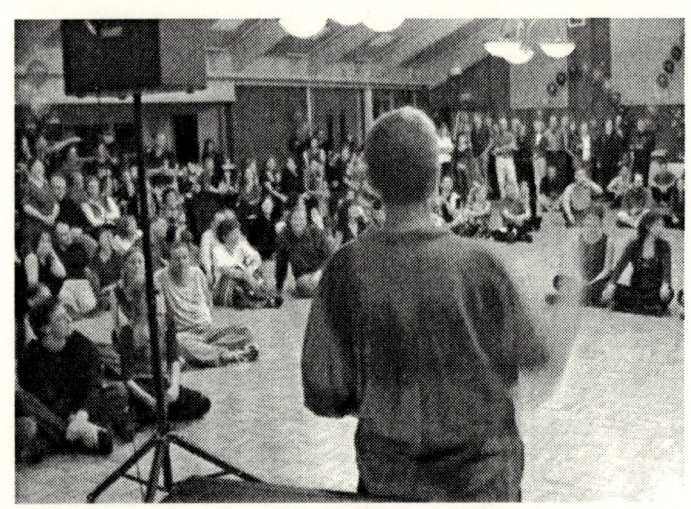

*I Talked*

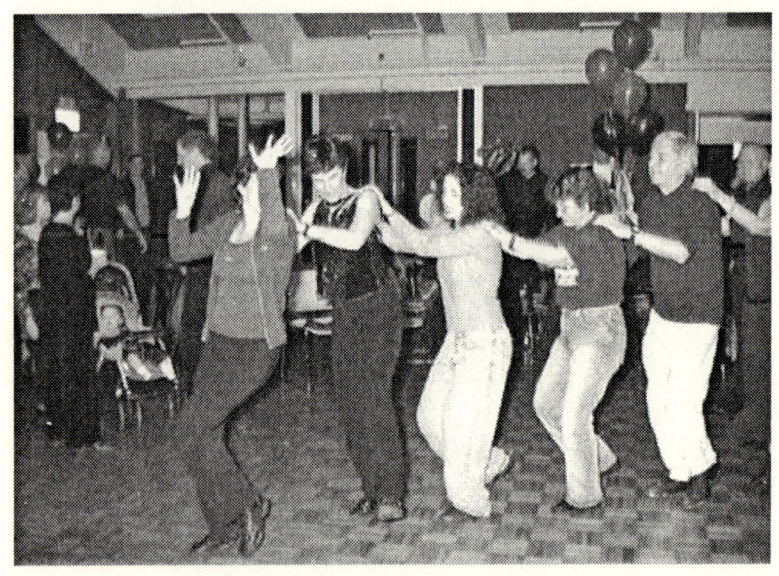

*And Then We Danced*

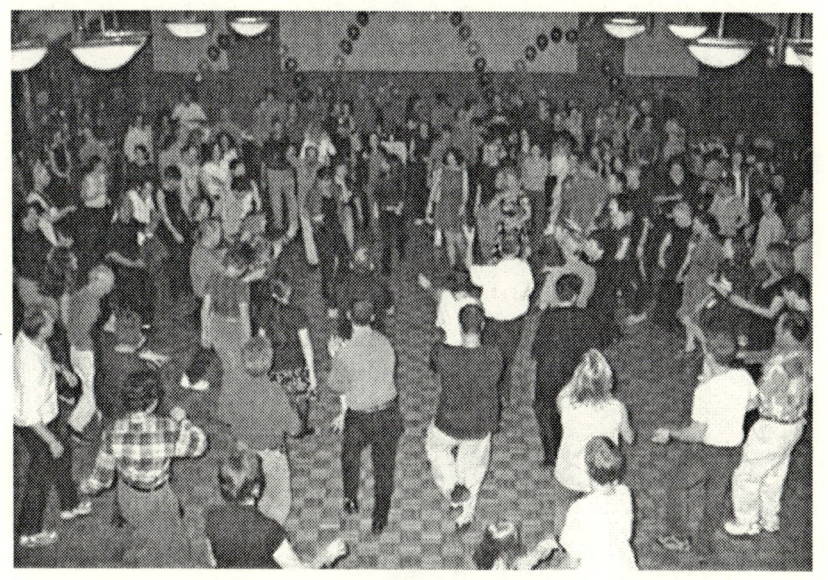

*And Danced!*

## Addendum (the words to the songs)

### "I Hope You Dance"

I hope you never lose your sense of wonder,
You get your fill to eat, but always keep that hunger,
May you never take one single breath for granted.
God forbid love ever leave you empty-handed.
I hope you still feel small when you stand beside the ocean,
Whenever one door closes, I hope one more opens.
Promise me that you'll give faith a fighting chance,
And when you get the choice to sit it out or dance.

I hope you dance…I hope you dance.

I hope you never fear those mountains in the distance,
Never settle for the path of least resistance.
Living might mean taking chances, but they're worth taking.
Loving might be a mistake but it's worth making.
Don't let some hell bent heart leave you bitter,
When you come close to selling out reconsider.
Give the heavens above more than just a passing glance,
And when you get the choice to sit it out or dance.

I hope you dance…I hope you dance.
I hope you dance…I hope you dance.

I hope you still feel small when you stand beside the ocean,
Whenever one door closes, I hope one more opens.
Promise me that you'll give faith a fighting chance,
And when you get the choice to sit it out or dance.

## Dancing with Cancer

Dance…I hope you dance.
I hope you dance…I hope you dance.
I hope you dance…I hope you dance..

\* \* \* \* \* \* \* \* \* \* \* \* \*

"Could I Have This Dance for the Rest of My Life?"

I'll always remember the song they were playing
The first time we danced and I knew.
As we swayed to the music and held to each other
I fell in love with you.

Could I have this dance for the rest of my life?
Would you be my partner every night?
When we're together it feels so right.
Could I have this dance for the rest of my life?

I'll always remember that magic moment
When I held you close to me.
As we moved together, I knew forever
You're all I'll ever need.

Could I have this dance for the rest of my life?
Would you be my partner every night?
When we're together it feels so right.
Could I have this dance for the rest of my life?

\* \* \* \* \* \* \* \* \* \* \* \* \*

# RADIATION REPORT

Sunday, January 19, 2003, 9:00 PM

I got some comments that, in last week's e-mail, I failed to say anything about my health and only wrote about The Big Celebration. Okay, I was on a sweet high and still glowing from all the love and energy that the party generated, and I forgot about my body for a bit. I'll bring you up to date.

Radiation has continued five days a week. The radiation staff has been wonderfully efficient. I leave my house at 8:00 AM, drive to the hospital, get the treatment, and am back in my car by 8:25 AM. The treatments themselves are painless. If anything is a bother, it's getting out of bed earlier than I'm used to.

I was scheduled for a total of 30 sessions, or rather 23 regular radiation sessions followed by 7 days of something called an electron boost. As of this past Friday the 17th, I have completed 21 sessions. Tomorrow, Monday, is a holiday, so my last two full radiation treatments will be Tuesday and Wednesday. Then I am scheduled to get the electron boost, which is a shorter but specific blast aimed directly at the site of the tumor.

I have quite a spectacular radiation burn on my left side, from my collarbone to just below my left breast, and laterally from the middle of my breast bone to just shy of my armpit. It's bright red and a bit blotchy. It is particularly fierce on my collarbone where the skin has dried and cracked. There is something similar going on around my left shoulder blade where the radiation exits my back. It's an area about the size of my hand, also bright red and blotchy, and the upper edge is cracked and dry.

It has been like getting a sunburn, having it start to peel, and getting another burn on top of that mess, over and over. Copious amounts of cortisone cream, aloe vera, and petroleum jelly keep it from itching too much. It is more unsightly than painful. I'm really only aware of the burns when I stretch or scrunch my shoulders.

So the abuse will be over this Wednesday, and I can start to heal. The electron boost is very site-specific and of such a short duration that most people don't burn from it. From what I've read, it takes several weeks for the radiated skin to get back to normal and even then the skin frequently feels different, a bit thicker and leathery. Oh well. Life goes on.

## PHOTOS OF THE PARTY

I've received one collection of photographs from David Bergen. I'm going to post them on several pages, so you can pick the ones you want to see. The page names should be self-explanatory. Enjoy!

www.louitucker.com/Partydecorations.htm
www.louitucker.com/Partydancing.htm
www.louitucker.com/Partypainting.htm
www.louitucker.com/Partytalking.htm
www.louitucker.com/PartyLouiandSabine.htm

## TAKING MY LEAVE

When I was in a therapy group back in the mid-80s, I remember how important it was to not just up and leave the group. Group members were required to give four weeks' notice of any plan to leave the group. The buzzwords at the time were "process" and "closure."

Now that I'm coming to the end of my cancer treatment and these Sunday writing sessions/e-mails will stop, I'm seeing how important it is for me to "get closure" and not just stop writing. I've become very attached to this process, just as I got attached to my group therapy and the women who attended. Am I going to feel lonely or liberated? Will I miss the connection or delight in the free time? I may continue to write and not send out what I write. I'll have to see how that feels. My plan right now is to write and send you what I write for the next two Sundays.

As I have said and written before, this connection has been a powerful force that contributed to my strength and sense of well-being, aided in my recovery, and lifted my heart. You may quibble if you wish, but I feel I have received far more than I have given.

"A good week, a week of peace
May gladness reign and joy increase"

Loui

\* \* \* \* \* \* \* \* \* \* \* \* \*

# JUST ONE MORE WEEK

## Sunday, January 26, 2003, 8:30 PM

Tuesday last week was my last day of three-blast radiation. On Wednesday, Thursday, and Friday, I only got the 50-second "electron boost," and I only have five more days of that. That also meant the skin on the left side of my chest and my left shoulder blade has had five days to heal. Even after these many months of chemotherapy and radiation, the body's ability to heal has not ceased to astonish me. The skin has gone from being an angry red to a sort of mildly annoyed red in that short period of time. There has been some peeling, which itches, but it has been no worse than your typical sunburn. By this time next week, I hope I won't need applications of cream three times a day.

To make sure the technicians aim the radiation machinery at the correct spot each time, the doctor drew around my very pale crescent-shaped scar, about a inch away all the way around. Drawing around a crescent shape gives you a blob-ish shape similar to a large lima bean. They don't put a tattoo for this procedure; they just use a marking pen and touch it up every day. I was cautioned not to wipe off the drawing, and I was asked to have someone touch it up over the weekend. That someone has been Sabine. Doesn't she have all the fun jobs around here?

I got a little silly last week and drew a happy face on my left breast, just to give the radiation technicians a giggle. I think the last Friday, I'll draw a little hand waving goodbye....

My hair has been a pleasant surprise. It is, as I wrote before, salt and pepper, with more salt than pepper. It appears to be slightly curly, or rather when I apply some gel and comb it up with my fingers, it curls a bit. It is all very amusing and entertaining after 50 years of straight-as-a-pin hair. I'm also finally seeing hair elsewhere on my body and am I relieved! The only place I've stayed "bald" is (surprise) my armpits—both sides, not just the side where the surgery was done.

## TRUSTING MY BODY

Way back in my 20s I remember having a wheel come off my car one night as I was driving home from a dance party. Really! It was not that I blew out a tire. I actually lost the back left wheel of my car and the entire thing—tire, hubcap, wheel, and bolts—all went bouncing away across the freeway. The empty metal axle hit the asphalt and sent a shower of sparks (I was on a freeway going 60 mph) like a rooster tail out behind the car. There wasn't much traffic and I was able to steer to the side of the road to safety.

After the repairs were made, it took me a month or two to completely trust my car again. I kept expecting some fatal light to flash on the dashboard or for something to suddenly fall off again. The car was fine, of course, and I drove it for several more years, but that one incident spooked me for quite a while.

I think I will probably feel the same way about my body after this brush with cancer. Whereas before, I viewed mammograms as an annoying and unnecessary interruption of my schedule, mammograms will take on a new and deeper significance for me. I won't put them off, and I won't treat them flippantly. A sore muscle will have me thinking "Cancer?" instead of "You overdid it again at the gym" or "Oops! Too much gardening this weekend." An unusual twinge or ache where there was no twinge or ache before will make me wonder if another tumor is growing inside me.

I wonder how long it will take before I can truly trust my body again.

## DEPRESSION? YOU'RE KIDDING, RIGHT?

To be honest, I was startled when one of you wrote me to be on the lookout for post-treatment depression. What a crazy idea! Then I did some reading and discovered that post-treatment depression does happen. Some cancer patients go through all the chemotherapy treatment and radiation with a great attitude and then succumb to depression when the treatment ends. They become accustomed to the routine of doctor visits and blood tests and getting care and advice from nurses and technicians. They get used to a constant stream of get-well wishes from everyone they encounter and people continually asking about their health and well-being. When they are done with the treatment and are in good health again, they miss all the attention!

I've been so relieved, so grateful, so elated that it's almost over, I cannot imagine being depressed. But then, what I could not imagine happening to me has already happened once—I got cancer. It doesn't hurt to be aware of the possibilities.

## THE END OF A CHAPTER

Something I remember from my therapist and my therapy group from the mid-1980s: 100% of all relationships end. Whether by your conscious decision or by the action of another or by death, all relationships end. They say the healthiest thing to do is mourn and move on.

While I was celebrating last weekend, I was rejoicing in reclaiming my body and my energy and my hair after a long, taxing struggle. Now I have to look at the end of this chapter as being the end of a special relationship with lots and lots of people (the last time I counted there were over 250 names in the e-mail group that receives these e-mails), and this relationship too has to end eventually. I've reconnected with old friends and strengthened existing ties. I've exchanged intimate details in writing with people I've never actually met. A lot of magical links were created during the past nine months. I hope the energy and linkage can continue even though I stop writing on a weekly basis.

Sundays evenings will be different for a while. I will fill the time with other activities, but I will remember what it was like to have a place for my emotions and feelings to go each week besides into the bits and bytes of computer software. I remember reading an interview with a comedian who said that "to have an audience is to be connected to a power source." That's what it's like, all right! Being connected to you all during this chapter of my life has been like being connected to a power source.

Five more days of radiation and I can close this book, pull the plug, and get on with the rest of my life.

Loui

* * * * * * * * * * * *

# THE END OF A CHAPTER

Sunday, February 2, 2003, 8:30 PM

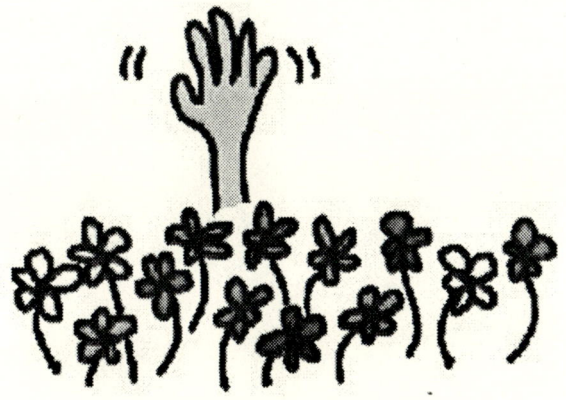

**TEN MONTHS (4/02–2/03)**

The end of a chapter
The closing of a door
The reaching of a goal

Turning the corner
Switching off the light
Arriving at the destination

The period at the end of a sentence
The flourish at the end of a dance
The curtain at the end of a scene
The last sweet notes of a song

Loui Tucker

One chapter leads to another
One door closes and another opens
One goal is reached and another beckons

Turn a corner and start down a new path
Switch off a light and the fun can begin
Arrive at a destination and start planning your next trip

Finish a sentence and keep on writing
This dance ends but the music doesn't stop
The curtain rises on another bright scene
One song ends and it's time to sing another

The challenge was met
The fears faced
The battle won
And Life goes on


Shalom,

Loui